Carnivore D

For Women Over 60

Transformative Nutrition Strategies For Women
Over 60 on the Carnivore Diet

Janet Cook

Copyright © 2023 by Janet Cook

All rights reserved. Except for brief quotations included in critical reviews and certain other noncommercial uses allowed by copyright law, no part of this publication may be reproduced, distributed, or transmitted in any form or by any means, including photocopying, recording, or other electronic or mechanical methods, without the publisher's prior written permission.

TABLE OF CONTENTS

INTRODUCTION: EMBRACING THE CARNIVORE DIET

CHAPTER ONE

CHAPTER TWO

BREAKFAST RECIPES

CLASSIC STEAK AND EGGS - A GUIDE TO PREPARING A TENDER STEAK WITH PERFECTLY COOKED EGGS.

PORK BELLY BREAKFAST BAKE - A HEARTY, OVEN-BAKED DISH.

LUNCH RECIPES

CLASSIC BEEF LIVER PATTIES WITH GARLIC AIOLI

CHICKEN CAESAR SALAD - A CARNIVORE TWIST ON A CLASSIC, USING HOMEMADE ANCHOVY DRESSING.

DINNER RECIPES

RIBEYE WITH BONE MARROW BUTTER - A LUXURIOUS MAIN COURSE.

DUCK BREAST WITH RED WINE REDUCTION - ELEGANT, WITH A FOCUS ON TECHNIQUE.

SLOW-COOKED PORK SHOULDER - A SIMPLE, VERSATILE RECIPE THAT CAN FEED YOU FOR DAYS.

SNACKS RECIPES

BEEF JERKY - HOMEMADE, NO ADDITIVES.

PORK RINDS - HOW TO PUFF AND SEASON AT HOME.

APPETIZERS RECIPES

TOP OF FORM SCALLOPS SEARED IN GHEE - LIGHT AND RICH IN FLAVOR.

Introduction: Embracing the Carnivore Diet

The Carnivore Diet, characterized by its exclusive focus on animal foods, has emerged as a fascinating and often controversial approach to nutrition and wellness. At its core, this diet simplifies eating by eliminating plant-based foods, concentrating instead on meats, fish, eggs, and certain dairy products. This guide aims to introduce women over 60 to the carnivore diet, highlighting its potential benefits and considerations specific to their nutritional needs and lifestyle.

Overview of the Carnivore Diet

The carnivore diet is rooted in the premise that human beings thrive on animal-based nutrition. Proponents argue that by focusing on high-quality animal products, individuals can achieve better health outcomes, including improved energy levels, weight management, and reduction of inflammation. This diet is not merely a high-protein intake plan but emphasizes the consumption of all parts of the animal, including organ meats and bone marrow, to maximize nutrient intake.

For women over 60, the carnivore diet offers particular advantages. This demographic often faces unique health challenges, such as hormonal changes, decreased bone density, and the need to preserve muscle mass. The nutrient density of animal products—rich in protein, vitamins, and minerals such as vitamin B12, iron, calcium, and zinc—can support these areas effectively. Furthermore, the diet's high protein content is crucial for maintaining muscle mass, which is essential for mobility, strength, and overall health.

Adopting a carnivore diet also simplifies meal planning and preparation. Without the need to consider fruits, vegetables, grains, or legumes, the focus shifts to quality and sourcing of animal products. This simplicity can be liberating, though it requires a mindful approach to ensure nutritional completeness.

Critics of the carnivore diet raise concerns about the lack of dietary fiber and potential risks associated with high intake of saturated fats and cholesterol. However, many who follow the diet report improvements in digestive issues, autoimmune conditions, and blood sugar regulation, suggesting that individual responses to dietary patterns can vary widely.

For women over 60 considering the carnivore diet, it is essential to approach this dietary shift with caution and awareness. Consulting with healthcare providers, paying attention to the body's signals, and choosing high-quality, ethically sourced animal products are critical steps in ensuring the diet's success and sustainability.

In conclusion, the carnivore diet presents a radical yet intriguing approach to nutrition that could offer significant health benefits, especially for women over 60. By focusing on nutrient-dense, animal-based foods, it is possible to support the body's needs effectively, promoting vitality and well-being in later life. As with any dietary change, it is crucial to undertake this journey with informed guidance, open-mindedness, and a commitment to health and happiness.

Benefits of the Carnivore Diet for Women Over 60: Hormonal Balance, Bone Density, and Muscle Preservation

For women over 60, maintaining optimal health becomes a priority, with specific focus areas such as hormonal balance, bone density, and muscle preservation. The carnivore diet, with its emphasis on high-quality animal proteins and fats, presents a compelling nutritional strategy to support these aspects of health. Here, we explore the benefits of adopting a carnivore diet for women in this age group, underlining its potential to enhance overall well-being.

Hormonal Balance

The post-menopausal years bring significant hormonal changes for women, often leading to symptoms like weight gain, mood fluctuations, and increased risk of certain diseases. The carnivore diet can play a pivotal role in stabilizing these hormonal shifts. High in fats and cholesterol, this diet provides essential components for hormone production, including estrogen and progesterone. By supplying the body with these crucial building blocks, women over 60 can experience improved hormonal balance, potentially mitigating some of the adverse effects associated with menopause.

Bone Density

Osteoporosis and decreased bone density are prevalent concerns for women over 60, attributed mainly to hormonal changes and calcium deficiency. The carnivore diet is rich in nutrients essential for bone health, including calcium, vitamin D, and phosphorus, found in dairy products, fish, and certain meats. Additionally, the high protein content of the diet supports the maintenance of bone mass. Studies suggest that dietary protein works synergistically with calcium to improve calcium absorption and bone metabolism, offering a protective effect against bone loss in older adults.

Muscle Preservation

Sarcopenia, or the age-related loss of muscle mass and function, poses a significant risk to the elderly, impacting mobility, strength, and independence. The carnivore diet, with its emphasis on protein, provides a robust foundation for combating muscle degradation. Adequate protein intake is critical for muscle protein synthesis, the process by which the body repairs and builds muscle tissue. The amino acids found in animal proteins are particularly effective in this regard, being highly bioavailable and complete in essential amino acids. Engaging in regular physical activity while following a carnivore diet can further enhance muscle preservation and strength, contributing to a better quality of life.

For women over 60, the carnivore diet offers a nutrient-dense approach to eating that aligns well with the body's changing needs. By focusing on animal-based foods, this diet provides key nutrients for hormonal balance, bone density, and muscle preservation. However, it's important to approach this diet with mindfulness, considering individual health conditions and consulting healthcare professionals to ensure it's the right choice. With the right precautions and a focus on high-quality, diverse animal foods, the carnivore diet can be a valuable tool in maintaining and enhancing health during the golden years.

Safely Transitioning to the Carnivore Diet for Women Over 60

Transitioning to a carnivore diet at any stage of life requires careful consideration, but for women over 60, it's especially important to ensure that the shift supports health without introducing unnecessary risks. The carnivore diet, focused entirely on animal products, may offer benefits like improved hormonal balance, bone density, and muscle preservation. However, a thoughtful approach is needed to transition safely and effectively. Here's a guide to help women over 60 navigate this change in their dietary habits.

1. Consult with Healthcare Professionals

Before making any significant dietary changes, consulting with a healthcare provider is crucial. This step is particularly important for women over 60, who may have specific health conditions or nutritional needs. A healthcare provider can offer personalized advice, considering your health history, current medications, and nutritional requirements. They can also help monitor your health as you transition to the diet.

2. Gradually Reduce Plant-Based Foods

A sudden shift to a carnivore diet can be a shock to the system. Instead, gradually reduce the intake of plant-based foods over several weeks. This gradual transition can help your body adjust to the new way of eating, minimizing potential digestive issues and allowing you to monitor how your body responds to each change.

3. Focus on Nutrient-Dense Animal Foods

Not all animal foods are created equal when it comes to nutrient density. Emphasize high-quality, nutrient-dense options such as organ meats, fatty fish, eggs, and grass-fed meats. These foods provide a wide range of nutrients critical for health, including vitamins B12, D, A, and essential minerals like iron, zinc, and selenium.

4. Monitor Nutrient Intake

While the carnivore diet can provide most of the nutrients needed for good health, there are potential gaps, such as fiber and certain vitamins found primarily in plants. Discuss with a healthcare provider or dietitian about how to monitor your nutrient intake and whether supplementation might be necessary, particularly for vitamins C and E, and fiber, if digestive health becomes a concern.

5. Stay Hydrated and Mindful of Electrolytes

Transitioning to a carnivore diet may affect your body's water and electrolyte balance. Ensure adequate hydration by drinking plenty of water. You may also need to pay attention to electrolyte intake, especially sodium, potassium, and magnesium, which are crucial for muscle function, nerve signaling, and overall health. Incorporating bone broths and considering electrolyte supplements can help maintain balance.

6. Listen to Your Body

As you transition, pay close attention to how your body responds. Some individuals may experience increased energy and improved health markers, while others may face challenges such as digestive changes or nutrient deficiencies. Adjustments may be necessary based on your body's feedback. Keep a journal of how you feel, what you eat, and any symptoms you experience to discuss with your healthcare provider.

7. Introduce Physical Activity

If not already part of your routine, incorporating physical activity can complement the benefits of a carnivore diet. Activities such as walking, strength training, and flexibility exercises can help maintain muscle mass, bone density, and overall well-being. Always consult with a healthcare provider before starting any new exercise regimen.

Transitioning to a carnivore diet for women over 60 offers a unique opportunity to address specific health concerns associated with aging. By taking a measured, mindful approach and consulting with healthcare professionals, it's possible to safely explore the benefits of this dietary change. Remember, individual experiences with the carnivore diet can vary, and it's essential to prioritize personal health and well-being throughout the transition process.

Important Nutritional Considerations for the Carnivore Diet

Adopting a carnivore diet means focusing exclusively on animal products. While this diet can provide high levels of certain nutrients, it requires careful planning to meet all of your body's nutritional needs. Here are key nutritional considerations for those on a carnivore diet and strategies to address them effectively.

1. Complete Protein

Consideration: Protein is crucial for muscle maintenance, hormone production, and overall health. Animal products offer complete proteins, containing all essential amino acids.

Strategy: Incorporate a variety of meats, including beef, chicken, fish, and eggs, to ensure a broad spectrum of amino acids. Including organ meats like liver can also provide a nutritional boost, offering not just protein but an array of vitamins and minerals.

2. Essential Fatty Acids

Consideration: Omega-3 and omega-6 fatty acids are essential for heart health, brain function, and reducing inflammation. Balancing these fats is crucial, as most people consume too many omega-6s and not enough omega-3s.

Strategy: Focus on fatty fish such as salmon, mackerel, and sardines, which are high in omega-3 fatty acids. Grass-fed meats and dairy can also have a more favorable omega-3 to omega-6 ratio compared to their grain-fed counterparts.

3. Vitamins and Minerals

Consideration: Certain vitamins and minerals that are abundant in plant foods might be consumed in lower amounts on a carnivore diet. These include vitamin C, vitamin E, and potentially some B vitamins.

Strategy: To address potential gaps in vitamin C, opt for fresh meats as cooking can reduce vitamin C content. Organ meats, especially liver, are rich in vitamins A, D, E, and K, as well as B vitamins. Consuming seafood can provide iodine and selenium, while dairy products can be a good source of calcium.

4. Bone Health

Consideration: Calcium is vital for bone health, and its primary sources in many diets are dairy products and fortified plant foods.

Strategy: Include dairy products in your diet, if tolerated, focusing on high-calcium options like cheese and yogurt. Bone broth, made from simmering bones for an extended period, can also provide calcium, magnesium, and phosphorus.

5. Electrolyte Balance

Consideration: A sudden shift to a carnivore diet can impact electrolyte levels, particularly during the initial adjustment period.

Strategy: Ensure adequate intake of sodium, potassium, and magnesium. While sodium is generally abundant in a carnivore diet, especially if you include processed meats, potassium can be found in meats, fish, and dairy. For magnesium, consider supplementation or consume specific fish like mackerel, which is higher in magnesium.

6. Hydration and Fiber

Consideration: The lack of dietary fiber in a carnivore diet can affect digestion and gut health for some individuals.

Strategy: Although traditional fiber sources are absent, many people on a carnivore diet report regular digestive function. Ensure adequate hydration to support digestive health. Some individuals may include a small amount of dairy, like cheese, which can provide some form of fermentable fiber for gut bacteria.

Adopting a carnivore diet requires mindful consideration of your nutritional intake to ensure your body receives the essential nutrients it needs. By focusing on a variety of high-quality animal products and being attentive to the unique nutritional challenges posed by this diet, individuals can effectively meet their nutritional requirements. Regular health check-ups and blood work can help monitor nutritional status and adjust the diet as necessary to maintain optimal health.

CHAPTER ONE

Getting Started - Understanding Your Nutritional Needs: Macros and Micros

Embarking on a dietary journey, such as adopting a carnivore diet, necessitates a foundational understanding of nutritional needs. This understanding ensures that your diet is balanced, fulfilling, and tailored to support your health goals and lifestyle. For individuals, especially women over 60, focusing on macro and micronutrient intake is crucial for maintaining vitality, muscle mass, and bone health. This section delves into the essentials of macronutrients (macros) and micronutrients (micros), providing a roadmap to navigate your nutritional needs effectively.

Understanding Macronutrients

Macronutrients are the primary components of our diet, providing energy and playing essential roles in body function and health. They include proteins, fats, and carbohydrates. On a carnivore diet, the focus is predominantly on proteins and fats, with minimal to no carbohydrates.

- **Proteins:** Essential for repairing tissues, building muscles, and producing enzymes and hormones. Proteins are made up of amino acids, some of which are essential because the body cannot produce them. Animal products provide complete proteins, containing all essential amino acids in optimal ratios.

- **Fats:** Serve as a major energy source, support cell growth, and aid in the absorption of certain vitamins. Fats also play a crucial role in hormone production, which is particularly important for post-menopausal women. Saturated and monounsaturated fats, found abundantly in animal products, are vital for brain health and energy.

- **Carbohydrates:** Generally excluded or minimized in a carnivore diet, carbohydrates are the body's primary energy source in traditional diets. However, the body can adapt to using fats for energy through a process called ketosis.

Understanding Micronutrients

Micronutrients, while required in smaller amounts than macronutrients, are vital for good health, supporting a range of bodily functions from bone health to immune response.

- **Vitamins:** Organic compounds that are crucial for metabolism, vision, and skin health, among other functions. Key vitamins for women over 60 include Vitamin D for bone health and immune function, Vitamin B12 for nerve function and energy production, and Vitamin A for vision and immune health.

- **Minerals:** Inorganic elements that play roles in bone health, cardiovascular health, and more. Important minerals include calcium for bone health, iron for blood production (though less of a concern post-menopause), and magnesium for muscle function and nervous system regulation.

Meeting Your Nutritional Needs on a Carnivore Diet

- **Protein and Fats:** Prioritize a variety of animal products, including muscle meats, organ meats, eggs, and fatty fish, to cover both your macro and micronutrient needs. Organ meats are particularly nutrient-dense, offering a concentrated source of vitamins and minerals.

- **Vitamins:** Ensure adequate intake of fat-soluble vitamins (A, D, E, and K) through fatty meats, fish, and organ meats. B vitamins are abundantly available in animal products, while Vitamin C, though lower in a carnivore diet, is present in fresh meats and organ meats.

- **Minerals:** Consume a variety of meats to ensure a broad intake of minerals. Bone broths and dairy (if included) can help meet calcium needs, while shellfish and organ meats can provide zinc and selenium.

Adopting a carnivore diet requires careful consideration of both macro and micronutrient needs to ensure a balanced and health-supportive eating plan. By focusing on nutrient-dense animal products and understanding the roles of various nutrients in the body, individuals can tailor their diet to support their health goals effectively. Regular monitoring and adjustments, guided by healthcare professionals, can ensure that nutritional needs are met, supporting vitality and health through the golden years.

Kitchen Essentials: Tools and Tips for Carnivore Cooking

Embarking on a carnivore diet journey brings a shift in kitchen dynamics, where the preparation of animal-based foods becomes the centerpiece of your culinary practice. This transition not only simplifies meal planning but also elevates the importance of having the right tools and techniques at your disposal. For women over 60, mastering the art of carnivore cooking can enhance the enjoyment and nutritional value of meals, making every bite both satisfying and nourishing. Here's a guide to the essential kitchen tools and tips for adeptly navigating carnivore cooking.

Essential Kitchen Tools

1. **High-Quality Knives:** A sharp, durable chef's knife and a sturdy boning knife are indispensable for efficiently cutting, trimming, and preparing meat. Investing in high-quality knives ensures precision in meal prep and can make cooking more enjoyable and less laborious.

2. **Cast Iron Skillet:** Ideal for searing and roasting, a cast iron skillet provides even heat distribution and enhances the flavor of meats. Its versatility allows for everything from cooking steaks to baking frittatas, making it a carnivore kitchen staple.

3. **Meat Thermometer:** Ensuring meats are cooked to the correct temperature is crucial for both safety and quality. A digital meat thermometer can help achieve the perfect doneness, whether you prefer your steak rare or well-done.

4. **Slow Cooker or Pressure Cooker:** These appliances are excellent for tenderizing tougher cuts of meat and making bone broth, a carnivore diet essential. They offer the convenience of set-it-and-forget-it cooking, ideal for busy or low-energy days.

5. **Cutting Board:** A large, sturdy cutting board made of wood or plastic is essential for handling and preparing large cuts of meat. Consider having separate boards for raw meats and other foods to maintain hygiene.

6. **Meat Tenderizer or Mallet:** Useful for tenderizing tougher cuts of meat, a meat tenderizer can help improve texture and reduce cooking time, making meats more palatable and easier to digest.

Tips for Carnivore Cooking

1. **Master the Art of Searing:** Learning to properly sear meat can transform your dishes. High heat for a short time creates a delicious crust while keeping

the inside tender and juicy. Remember to pat your meat dry and let it come to room temperature for even cooking.

2. **Rest Your Meat:** Allowing meat to rest after cooking before cutting into it helps retain its juices, ensuring your dish is moist and flavorful. The resting time depends on the size of the cut but generally ranges from 5 to 15 minutes.

3. **Utilize Leftovers:** Creativity with leftovers can simplify your carnivore diet. Leftover meats can be repurposed into salads, omelets, or broths, reducing waste and saving time.

4. **Experiment with Marinades and Rubs:** While a carnivore diet focuses on animal products, certain spices and seasonings can be used to enhance flavor. Experiment with simple rubs and marinades that align with your dietary preferences to add variety to your meals.

5. **Invest in Quality:** Whenever possible, choose high-quality, grass-fed, and organic meats. These options tend to be more nutrient-dense and ethically sourced, supporting both your health and the environment.

Setting up your kitchen with essential tools and embracing useful cooking tips can significantly enhance your experience on the carnivore diet. These essentials and techniques not only streamline the cooking process but also ensure that your meals are delicious, nutritious, and satisfying. As you become more comfortable and creative in your carnivore cooking journey, you'll discover the joy and simplicity in preparing meals that nourish both the body and soul.

Shopping Guide: Choosing the Best Meats and Animal Products

For individuals embarking on a carnivore diet, particularly women over 60, selecting high-quality meats and animal products is paramount. The quality of the meat not only impacts the flavor and enjoyment of your meals but also affects your overall health and nutrition. This comprehensive guide will walk you through the essentials of choosing the best meats and animal products, ensuring that your carnivore diet is both nourishing and satisfying.

Understanding Meat Quality

1. **Grass-Fed vs. Grain-Fed:** Grass-fed animals are raised on a natural diet of grass, which can lead to meat that's higher in certain nutrients, including omega-3 fatty acids and antioxidants. Grain-fed animals are often raised in feedlots with a diet designed to fatten them quickly, possibly affecting the nutritional quality and taste of the meat.

2. **Organic:** Organic meats come from animals that are not given antibiotics or hormones and are raised on organic feed. Choosing organic can reduce your exposure to residues from pesticides and potentially harmful chemicals.

3. **Pasture-Raised:** This term indicates animals were raised in a more natural environment, allowed to graze and roam. Pasture-raised animals generally enjoy a better quality of life and produce meat that could be leaner and richer in certain vitamins.

Selecting Specific Meats and Products

1. **Beef:** Look for grass-fed and organic labels to ensure you're getting beef that is not only better for you but also has a superior taste. Pay attention to marbling – the fat within the muscle – for more flavorful and tender cuts.

2. **Poultry:** Free-range or pasture-raised poultry is preferable. These birds have access to the outdoors, which contributes to a better nutritional profile, including higher vitamin D content.

3. **Pork:** Similar to beef, look for pasture-raised or organic pork. These pigs have a varied diet and more humane living conditions, affecting the taste and quality of the meat.

4. **Fish:** Opt for wild-caught fish over farmed to avoid potential contaminants and to benefit from a higher nutrient content. Look for sustainable certifications to ensure the fishery is managed in a

way that preserves the species and the environment.

5. **Eggs:** Choose pasture-raised eggs when possible. These eggs come from hens that roam freely and have a diet that results in eggs richer in omega-3 fatty acids and vitamins.

6. **Dairy:** For those who include dairy in their carnivore diet, select full-fat, grass-fed dairy products. These are higher in omega-3s and fat-soluble vitamins. Raw dairy products may offer additional benefits, but make sure they are from a reputable source to avoid health risks.

Tips for Shopping

1. **Local Farmers Markets:** Shopping at farmers markets can provide access to fresh, local meat and animal products. It also offers the opportunity to speak directly with farmers about their practices.

2. **Butcher Shops:** A knowledgeable butcher can provide advice on the best cuts for your needs and offer insight into the sourcing of their meats.

3. **Bulk Purchases:** Consider buying meat in bulk directly from a farm or butcher. This can be cost-effective and ensures you have a supply of high-

quality meat. Many farms offer "shares" of animals that include a variety of cuts.

4. **Online Suppliers:** There are many reputable online suppliers of high-quality meats and animal products. This can be a convenient option to access grass-fed, organic, or specialty meats not available locally.

5. **Label Reading:** Always read labels carefully. Terms like "natural" can be misleading and don't guarantee the meat meets the higher standards of organic or grass-fed.

Choosing the right meats and animal products is crucial for anyone following a carnivore diet, especially for women over 60 looking to maximize health benefits. By focusing on quality, such as grass-fed, organic, and pasture-raised options, you can ensure your diet is rich in essential nutrients and free from unnecessary additives. Educating yourself on the best practices for selecting meats and staying informed about where and how your food is produced will empower you to make choices that support your health and dietary goals.

CHAPTER TWO

Breakfast Recipes

Classic Steak and Eggs - A guide to preparing a tender steak with perfectly cooked eggs.

Classic Steak and Eggs Recipe

Recipe 1: Herb-Butter Steak and Sunny-Side Up Eggs

Prep	**Time:**	10	minutes
Cook	**Time:**	15	minutes
Total	**Time:**	25	minutes

Servings: 2

Ingredients:

- 2 ribeye steaks (approx. 8 oz each)
- 4 large eggs
- 2 tablespoons unsalted butter, softened
- 1 tablespoon fresh parsley, finely chopped
- 1 teaspoon fresh thyme, finely chopped
- Salt and freshly ground black pepper, to taste
- 2 tablespoons olive oil

Instructions:

1. **Prepare the Herb Butter:** In a small bowl, mix together the softened butter, parsley, thyme, salt, and pepper. Set aside.

2. **Cook the Steak:** Season the steaks generously with salt and pepper. Heat 1 tablespoon of olive oil in a cast-iron skillet over medium-high heat. Add the steaks and cook for about 4-5 minutes on each side for medium-rare, or until desired doneness. Remove steaks from the skillet and let them rest for 5 minutes.

3. **Cook the Eggs:** In the same skillet, reduce heat to medium. Add the remaining olive oil. Crack the eggs into the skillet, being careful not to break the yolks. Cook for 2-3 minutes or until the whites are set but the yolks are still runny. Season with salt and pepper.

4. **Serve:** Slice the steak against the grain. Top each steak with a dollop of herb butter. Serve with sunny-side-up eggs on the side.

Nutritional Information (per serving):

- Calories: 620

- Protein: 52g

- Fat: 44g
- Carbohydrates: 1g
- Cholesterol: 400mg
- Sodium: 220mg

Chef's Tips:

- Let the steak come to room temperature for about 20 minutes before cooking to ensure even cooking.
- For extra flavor, baste the steak with the herb butter while it rests.
- Use fresh herbs for the butter to maximize the flavor profile.

Recipe 2: Seared Steak and Scrambled Eggs with Avocado

Prep Time: 5 minutes
Cook Time: 10 minutes
Total Time: 15 minutes
Servings: 2

Ingredients:

- 2 New York strip steaks (approx. 6 oz each)
- 6 large eggs
- 1/4 cup heavy cream
- 2 tablespoons unsalted butter
- 1 ripe avocado, sliced
- Salt and freshly ground black pepper, to taste
- 1 tablespoon olive oil

Instructions:

1. **Prepare the Eggs:** In a bowl, whisk together the eggs, heavy cream, salt, and pepper until well combined.
2. **Cook the Steak:** Season the steaks with salt and pepper. Heat the olive oil in a skillet over medium-

high heat. Add the steaks and cook for about 3-4 minutes on each side for medium-rare, or to your preferred doneness. Remove from the skillet and let rest.

3. **Scramble the Eggs:** Reduce heat to low. Melt butter in the same skillet. Add the egg mixture and gently stir for 2-3 minutes, or until the eggs are softly set. Remove from heat immediately to avoid overcooking.

4. **Serve:** Slice the rested steaks against the grain. Serve alongside scrambled eggs and top with sliced avocado.

Nutritional Information (per serving):

- Calories: 590
- Protein: 49g
- Fat: 42g
- Carbohydrates: 6g
- Cholesterol: 390mg
- Sodium: 210mg

Chef's Tips:

- Whisking a bit of heavy cream into the eggs before cooking them can make the scrambled eggs more luxurious and fluffy.

- Resting the steak after cooking is crucial for retaining its juices and ensuring it's moist and tender.

- Adding avocado not only provides healthy fats but also a creamy texture that complements the richness of the eggs and steak.

Pork Belly Breakfast Bake

Prep Time: 15 minutes
Cook Time: 1 hour 30 minutes
Total Time: 1 hour 45 minutes
Servings: 4

Ingredients:

- 1 lb pork belly, skin removed and cut into ½-inch cubes

- 8 large eggs

- ½ cup heavy cream

- 1 tablespoon olive oil

- Salt and freshly ground black pepper, to taste
- 1 teaspoon smoked paprika
- ¼ cup green onions, chopped for garnish

Instructions:

1. **Preheat the Oven:** Preheat your oven to 375°F (190°C).

2. **Cook the Pork Belly:** In a large ovenproof skillet, heat the olive oil over medium heat. Add the pork belly cubes and season with salt, pepper, and smoked paprika. Cook until the pork belly is crispy and golden brown, about 8-10 minutes. Remove from the heat and spread the pork belly evenly across the bottom of the skillet.

3. **Prepare the Egg Mixture:** In a mixing bowl, whisk together the eggs, heavy cream, salt, and pepper. Pour the egg mixture over the crispy pork belly in the skillet.

4. **Bake:** Transfer the skillet to the oven and bake for 25-30 minutes, or until the eggs are set and the top is lightly golden.

5. **Serve:** Let the breakfast bake cool slightly before slicing. Garnish with chopped green onions before serving.

Nutritional Information (per serving):

- Calories: 710
- Protein: 24g
- Fat: 65g
- Carbohydrates: 2g
- Cholesterol: 425mg
- Sodium: 320mg

Chef's Tips:

- For an extra crispy pork belly, pat the cubes dry before seasoning and cooking.
- Letting the bake rest for a few minutes after removing it from the oven will make it easier to slice and serve.

Beef Liver Patties with Aiolis

Prep Time: 20 minutes
Cook Time: 10 minutes
Total Time: 30 minutes
Servings: 4

Ingredients:

- 1 lb beef liver, finely minced
- 2 large eggs, beaten
- ½ cup almond flour
- 1 onion, finely chopped
- 2 cloves garlic, minced
- Salt and freshly ground black pepper, to taste
- 2 tablespoons olive oil
- For the Aioli:
    - ½ cup mayonnaise
    - 1 clove garlic, minced
    - 1 tablespoon lemon juice
    - Salt and pepper, to taste

Instructions:

1. **Prepare the Liver Mixture:** In a large bowl, combine the minced beef liver, beaten eggs, almond flour, chopped onion, minced garlic, salt, and pepper. Mix until well combined.

2. **Form Patties:** Shape the mixture into small patties, about ½ inch thick.

3. **Cook Patties:** Heat the olive oil in a skillet over medium heat. Cook the patties for about 4-5 minutes on each side, or until they are golden brown and cooked through.

4. **Prepare the Aioli:** While the patties are cooking, mix together mayonnaise, minced garlic, lemon juice, salt, and pepper in a small bowl. Adjust the seasoning to taste.

5. **Serve:** Serve the beef liver patties hot with a dollop of aioli on top or on the side for dipping.

Nutritional Information (per serving):

- Calories: 460
- Protein: 27g
- Fat: 35g

- Carbohydrates: 8g

- Cholesterol: 380mg

- Sodium: 300mg

Chef's Tips:

- Soaking the minced beef liver in milk for an hour before cooking can help mellow the flavor for those sensitive to the taste of liver.

- Ensure not to overcrowd the skillet when cooking the patties to allow them to get a good sear and prevent steaming.

- The aioli can be made in advance and stored in the refrigerator to allow the flavors to meld together.

Salmon Avocado Boats - Nutrient-rich start with omega-3 fatty acids (note: for those who include fish and avocados in their carnivore diet).

Smoked Salmon Avocado Boats with Poached Eggs

Prep Time: 10 minutes
Cook Time: 5 minutes
Total Time: 15 minutes
Servings: 2

Ingredients:

- 1 ripe avocado, halved and pit removed
- 4 oz smoked salmon
- 2 large eggs
- 1 tablespoon white vinegar
- Salt and freshly ground black pepper, to taste
- Fresh dill for garnish

Instructions:

1. **Prepare the Avocado:** Carefully scoop out a bit of the avocado flesh to create more space. Chop the removed flesh and set aside.

2. **Poach the Eggs:** Bring a pot of water to a simmer and add the white vinegar. Crack an egg into a small bowl and gently slide it into the simmering water. Repeat with the second egg. Poach for 3-4 minutes or until the whites are set but yolks are

still runny. Remove with a slotted spoon and drain on a paper towel.

3. **Assemble the Boats:** Place the smoked salmon inside the hollowed-out avocados. Add the chopped avocado on top of the salmon.

4. **Top with Poached Eggs:** Place a poached egg on each avocado boat. Season with salt and pepper, and garnish with fresh dill.

5. **Serve:** Enjoy immediately for a fresh and nutritious start to your day.

Nutritional Information (per serving):

- Calories: 320
- Protein: 19g
- Fat: 23g
- Carbohydrates: 9g (Net Carbs: 2g)
- Cholesterol: 185mg
- Sodium: 670mg

Chef's Tips:

- Use avocados that are ripe but still firm to make it easier to handle and fill.

- For perfectly poached eggs, create a gentle whirlpool in the simmering water before adding the egg to help the white wrap around the yolk.

- Smoked salmon can be substituted with cooked, flaked salmon for a different texture and flavor profile.

Baked Salmon Avocado Boats with Crispy Bacon

Prep Time: 5 minutes
Cook Time: 15 minutes
Total Time: 20 minutes
Servings: 2

Ingredients:

- 1 ripe avocado, halved and pit removed
- 4 oz fresh salmon fillet
- 4 slices of bacon, cooked and crumbled
- Salt and freshly ground black pepper, to taste
- Lemon wedges for serving
- Fresh chives, chopped for garnish

Instructions:

1. **Preheat the Oven:** Preheat your oven to 350°F (175°C).

2. **Prepare the Salmon:** Season the salmon fillet with salt and pepper. Place on a baking sheet and bake for 12-15 minutes, or until cooked through and flaky.

3. **Prepare the Avocado:** While the salmon is cooking, scoop out a bit of the avocado flesh to create more space if needed.

4. **Assemble the Boats:** Once the salmon is cooked, flake it with a fork and divide it among the avocado halves. Top with crumbled bacon.

5. **Bake the Avocado Boats:** Place the filled avocado halves back in the oven and bake for an additional 5 minutes.

6. **Serve:** Garnish with fresh chives and serve with lemon wedges on the side.

Nutritional Information (per serving):

- Calories: 400
- Protein: 24g
- Fat: 32g
- Carbohydrates: 9g (Net Carbs: 2g)
- Cholesterol: 55mg
- Sodium: 760mg

Chef's Tips:

- Cooking the bacon until crispy provides a delightful texture contrast to the creamy avocado and tender salmon.
- Squeezing lemon over the avocado boats before serving adds a burst of freshness that complements the fatty richness of the salmon and avocado.
- For an extra kick of flavor, consider adding a sprinkle of smoked paprika or chili flakes before baking the avocado boats.

Lemon Herb Salmon Avocado Boats

Prep Time: 10 minutes
Cook Time: 20 minutes
Total Time: 30 minutes
Servings: 2

Ingredients:

- 1 ripe avocado, halved and pit removed
- 4 oz salmon fillet
- 1 tablespoon olive oil
- 1 tablespoon lemon juice
- 1 teaspoon fresh dill, chopped
- 1 teaspoon fresh parsley, chopped
- Salt and freshly ground black pepper, to taste
- Lemon slices for garnish

Instructions:

1. **Preheat the Oven:** Preheat your oven to 375°F (190°C).
2. **Marinate the Salmon:** In a small bowl, mix together olive oil, lemon juice, dill, parsley, salt, and pepper. Place the salmon fillet in a baking

dish, and pour the marinade over it. Let it marinate for about 10 minutes.

3. **Bake the Salmon:** Place the baking dish in the oven and bake the salmon for 12-15 minutes, or until it flakes easily with a fork.

4. **Prepare the Avocado:** While the salmon is baking, prepare the avocado halves by scooping out a little of the flesh to make room for the salmon. You can dice the scooped-out avocado and set it aside for topping.

5. **Assemble the Boats:** Once the salmon is done, break it into flakes and divide it among the avocado halves. Top with the diced avocado.

6. **Serve:** Garnish with lemon slices and additional fresh herbs if desired. Serve immediately.

Nutritional Information (per serving):

- Calories: 345
- Protein: 23g
- Fat: 26g
- Carbohydrates: 9g (Net Carbs: 2g)
- Cholesterol: 55mg

- Sodium: 125mg

Chef's Tips:

- Letting the salmon marinate, even for a short time, infuses it with flavor. You can prepare the marinade ahead of time for a deeper flavor.

- Use a preheated oven to ensure even cooking of the salmon.

- The addition of fresh lemon juice not only adds a zesty flavor but also enhances the absorption of omega-3 fatty acids.

Spicy Grilled Salmon Avocado Boats

Prep Time: 15 minutes
Cook Time: 10 minutes
Total Time: 25 minutes
Servings: 2

Ingredients:

- 1 ripe avocado, halved and pit removed
- 4 oz salmon fillet
- 1 tablespoon olive oil
- 1 teaspoon chili powder
- 1/2 teaspoon garlic powder
- Salt and freshly ground black pepper, to taste
- Fresh cilantro for garnish
- Lime wedges for serving

Instructions:

1. **Preheat the Grill:** Preheat your grill to medium-high heat.
2. **Season the Salmon:** Rub the salmon fillet with olive oil and season with chili powder, garlic powder, salt, and pepper.

3. **Grill the Salmon:** Place the salmon on the grill, skin-side down. Grill for about 5-6 minutes on one side, then flip and grill for another 3-4 minutes, or until the salmon is cooked through and flakes easily.

4. **Prepare the Avocado:** While the salmon is grilling, prepare the avocado halves by scooping out a little of the flesh to make room for the salmon. You can chop the scooped-out avocado and set it aside for topping.

5. **Assemble the Boats:** Once the salmon is grilled, flake it with a fork and divide it among the avocado halves. Top with the chopped avocado.

6. **Serve:** Garnish with fresh cilantro and serve with lime wedges on the side. The lime juice adds a refreshing contrast to the spicy salmon.

Nutritional Information (per serving):

- Calories: 350
- Protein: 24g
- Fat: 27g
- Carbohydrates: 9g (Net Carbs: 2g)
- Cholesterol: 60mg

- Sodium: 200mg

Chef's Tips:

- Grilling the salmon not only adds a smoky flavor but also creates a delightful texture contrast with the creamy avocado.

- Adjust the level of spiciness to your preference by increasing or decreasing the amount of chili powder.

- Serving with lime not only enhances flavors but also adds a refreshing zest, balancing the richness of the salmon and avocado.

Pork Belly Breakfast Bake - A hearty, oven-baked dish.

Cheesy Pork Belly Breakfast Bake

Prep Time: 15 minutes
Cook Time: 35 minutes
Total Time: 50 minutes
Servings: 4

Ingredients:

- 1 lb pork belly, cut into ½-inch cubes
- 6 large eggs
- ½ cup heavy cream
- 1 cup shredded cheddar cheese
- 2 tablespoons unsalted butter
- Salt and freshly ground black pepper, to taste
- 1/4 cup green onions, chopped for garnish

Instructions:

1. **Preheat the Oven:** Preheat your oven to 375°F (190°C).

2. **Brown the Pork Belly:** In a large skillet over medium heat, melt the butter and add the pork belly cubes. Season with salt and pepper. Cook until the pork belly is crispy and golden, about 8-10 minutes. Transfer to a greased baking dish.

3. **Mix Eggs and Cream:** In a bowl, whisk together the eggs and heavy cream. Season with a pinch of salt and pepper.

4. **Assemble the Bake:** Pour the egg mixture over the crispy pork belly in the baking dish. Sprinkle shredded cheddar cheese evenly on top.

5. **Bake:** Bake in the preheated oven for 25-30 minutes, or until the eggs are set and the cheese is bubbly and golden.

6. **Serve:** Let the bake cool for a few minutes, then garnish with chopped green onions before serving.

Nutritional Information (per serving):

- Calories: 720
- Protein: 29g

- Fat: 65g
- Carbohydrates: 2g
- Cholesterol: 385mg
- Sodium: 320mg

Chef's Tips:

- For a lighter version, substitute half of the heavy cream with whole milk.
- Letting the pork belly rest on paper towels after cooking will remove excess fat, making the dish less greasy.
- This dish can be prepared ahead and refrigerated overnight before baking, making your morning routine easier.

Spicy Pork Belly and Egg Breakfast Bake

Prep Time: 20 minutes
Cook Time: 40 minutes
Total Time: 1 hour
Servings: 4

Ingredients:

- 1 lb pork belly, cut into ½-inch cubes
- 8 large eggs
- 1 jalapeño, finely diced
- ½ cup full-fat coconut milk
- 2 tablespoons olive oil
- 1 teaspoon cayenne pepper (adjust to taste)
- Salt and freshly ground black pepper, to taste
- Fresh cilantro, chopped for garnish

Instructions:

1. **Preheat the Oven:** Preheat your oven to 350°F (175°C).
2. **Cook the Pork Belly:** Heat olive oil in a skillet over medium heat. Add the pork belly cubes and season with salt, cayenne pepper, and black

pepper. Cook until the pork belly is crispy, about 10-12 minutes. Transfer to a baking dish.

3. **Prepare the Egg Mixture:** In a large bowl, whisk together the eggs, coconut milk, diced jalapeño, and a pinch of salt. Ensure it's well combined for a smooth consistency.

4. **Combine and Bake:** Pour the egg mixture over the cooked pork belly in the baking dish. Stir slightly to ensure the mixture is evenly distributed.

5. **Bake:** Place the dish in the preheated oven and bake for 30-35 minutes, or until the eggs are set and the top is slightly golden.

6. **Serve:** Allow the bake to cool for a few minutes. Garnish with fresh cilantro before serving.

Nutritional Information (per serving):

- Calories: 745
- Protein: 31g
- Fat: 68g
- Carbohydrates: 3g
- Cholesterol: 425mg
- Sodium: 330mg

Chef's Tips:

- Adjust the amount of cayenne pepper based on your preference for spice. Adding more will increase the heat, while less will make it milder.

- Coconut milk adds a unique flavor and creamy texture to the eggs, but it can be substituted with heavy cream if preferred.

- To ensure even cooking, cut the pork belly into uniform pieces. This promotes consistent crispiness and flavor in every bite.

Maple-Glazed Pork Belly Breakfast Bake

Prep Time: 20 minutes
Cook Time: 1 hour
Total Time: 1 hour 20 minutes
Servings: 4

Ingredients:

- 1 lb pork belly, cut into 1-inch cubes
- 6 large eggs
- 1/3 cup maple syrup
- 2 tablespoons apple cider vinegar
- 1 tablespoon Dijon mustard
- 1 teaspoon smoked paprika
- Salt and freshly ground black pepper, to taste
- 1/4 cup chopped parsley, for garnish

Instructions:

1. **Preheat the Oven:** Preheat your oven to 375°F (190°C).
2. **Marinate Pork Belly:** In a bowl, whisk together maple syrup, apple cider vinegar, Dijon mustard, smoked paprika, salt, and pepper. Toss the pork

belly cubes in the marinade until well coated. Let marinate for 15 minutes.

3. **Bake Pork Belly:** Spread the pork belly cubes on a baking sheet in a single layer. Bake for 25-30 minutes until the edges are crispy and caramelized.

4. **Prepare the Egg Mixture:** While the pork belly is baking, whisk together the eggs with a pinch of salt and pepper.

5. **Assemble the Bake:** Remove the pork belly from the oven and transfer to a baking dish. Pour the egg mixture over the pork belly. Stir slightly to ensure the mixture is well combined.

6. **Bake Again:** Place the baking dish back in the oven and bake for an additional 30 minutes, or until the eggs are set and the top is golden.

7. **Serve:** Allow the bake to cool for a few minutes before garnishing with chopped parsley. Serve warm.

Nutritional Information (per serving):

- Calories: 690
- Protein: 25g
- Fat: 58g

- Carbohydrates: 15g
- Cholesterol: 372mg
- Sodium: 320mg

    Chef's Tips:

- Marinating the pork belly not only infuses it with flavor but also helps to tenderize the meat.
- For a deeper flavor, consider adding a touch of ground cinnamon or nutmeg to the marinade.
- Ensure the pork belly cubes are spread out in a single layer during the initial bake for even caramelization.

Keto-Friendly Pork Belly and Mushroom Breakfast Bake

Prep Time: 15 minutes
Cook Time: 45 minutes
Total Time: 1 hour
Servings: 4

Ingredients:

- 1 lb pork belly, cut into ½-inch cubes
- 8 large eggs
- ½ cup heavy cream
- 1 cup sliced mushrooms
- 2 tablespoons olive oil
- 1 teaspoon garlic powder
- Salt and freshly ground black pepper, to taste
- Fresh thyme, for garnish

Instructions:

1. **Preheat the Oven:** Preheat your oven to 350°F (175°C).
2. **Sauté Mushrooms:** Heat 1 tablespoon of olive oil in a skillet over medium heat. Add the sliced

mushrooms and cook until they are soft and golden brown, about 5-7 minutes. Season with salt and pepper. Set aside.

3. **Cook Pork Belly:** In the same skillet, add the remaining olive oil and pork belly cubes. Season with garlic powder, salt, and pepper. Cook until the pork belly is crispy, about 10 minutes. Remove from heat.

4. **Prepare the Egg Mixture:** In a large bowl, whisk together the eggs and heavy cream. Season with a pinch of salt and pepper.

5. **Combine Ingredients:** In a baking dish, combine the cooked pork belly, sautéed mushrooms, and egg mixture. Stir slightly to distribute the ingredients evenly.

6. **Bake:** Place the baking dish in the preheated oven and bake for 35-40 minutes, or until the eggs are set and the top is slightly golden.

7. **Serve:** Let the bake rest for a few minutes before serving. Garnish with fresh thyme leaves.

Nutritional Information (per serving):

- Calories: 680
- Protein: 28g

- Fat: 62g
- Carbohydrates: 4g
- Cholesterol: 450mg
- Sodium: 320mg

Chef's Tips:

- Sautéing the mushrooms before adding them to the bake helps to release their moisture and concentrate their flavor.
- For a lighter version, substitute half of the heavy cream with unsweetened almond milk.
- Adding a variety of mushrooms can enhance the flavor and texture of the bake.

Lunch Recipes

Classic Beef Liver Patties with Garlic Aioli

Prep Time: 20 minutes
Cook Time: 10 minutes
Total Time: 30 minutes
Servings: 4

Ingredients:

For the Patties:

- 1 lb beef liver, finely minced
- 1 medium onion, finely chopped
- 2 cloves garlic, minced
- 2 large eggs
- 1/2 cup almond flour
- Salt and freshly ground black pepper, to taste
- 2 tablespoons olive oil, for frying

For the Garlic Aioli:

- 1/2 cup mayonnaise
- 2 cloves garlic, minced

- 1 tablespoon lemon juice
- Salt and pepper, to taste

Instructions:

1. **Prepare the Patties:** In a large bowl, combine minced beef liver, chopped onion, minced garlic, eggs, and almond flour. Season with salt and pepper, and mix until well combined.

2. **Form Patties:** Shape the mixture into small patties, about 1/2 inch thick.

3. **Cook Patties:** Heat olive oil in a large skillet over medium heat. Fry the patties for about 4-5 minutes on each side, or until they are golden brown and cooked through.

4. **Make the Garlic Aioli:** While the patties are cooking, prepare the aioli by mixing mayonnaise, minced garlic, lemon juice, salt, and pepper in a small bowl until smooth.

5. **Serve:** Serve the beef liver patties hot with a dollop of garlic aioli on top.

Nutritional Information (per serving):

- Calories: 405
- Protein: 27g
- Fat: 29g
- Carbohydrates: 9g
- Cholesterol: 380mg
- Sodium: 320mg

Chef's Tips:

- Soaking the beef liver in milk for a few hours before cooking can help reduce its strong flavor. Just make sure to pat it dry before mincing.
- Ensure the skillet is hot before adding the patties to get a nice sear on the outside while keeping the inside tender.
- The garlic aioli can be prepared in advance and stored in the refrigerator to allow the flavors to meld together more fully.

Herbed Beef Liver Patties with Rosemary Aioli

Prep Time: 15 minutes
Cook Time: 10 minutes
Total Time: 25 minutes
Servings: 4

Ingredients:

For the Patties:

- 1 lb beef liver, finely minced
- 1/2 cup breadcrumbs (for a carnivore diet, substitute with crushed pork rinds)
- 1 small onion, grated
- 2 tablespoons fresh parsley, chopped
- 1 tablespoon fresh thyme, chopped
- 2 eggs, beaten
- Salt and freshly ground black pepper, to taste
- 4 tablespoons butter, for frying

For the Rosemary Aioli:

- 1/2 cup mayonnaise
- 1 teaspoon fresh rosemary, finely chopped

- 1 clove garlic, minced
- 2 teaspoons Dijon mustard
- 1 tablespoon olive oil
- Salt and pepper, to taste

Instructions:

1. **Prepare the Patties:** In a bowl, combine the minced beef liver, breadcrumbs (or pork rind crumbs for a pure carnivore option), grated onion, parsley, thyme, and beaten eggs. Season with salt and pepper, and mix until well combined.

2. **Form Patties:** Shape the mixture into 4 large patties or 8 smaller ones, depending on your preference.

3. **Cook Patties:** Melt butter in a skillet over medium heat. Cook the patties for 3-4 minutes on each side, or until they are nicely browned and cooked through.

4. **Make the Rosemary Aioli:** Combine mayonnaise, rosemary, minced garlic, Dijon mustard, and olive oil in a small bowl. Season with salt and pepper to taste and whisk until smooth.

5. **Serve:** Arrange the beef liver patties on plates and top or serve with the rosemary aioli.

Nutritional Information (per serving):

- Calories: 450
- Protein: 28g
- Fat: 34g
- Carbohydrates: 11g (if using pork rinds, carbs will be lower)
- Cholesterol: 385mg
- Sodium: 330mg

Chef's Tips:

- If using pork rinds as a breadcrumb substitute, ensure they are finely crushed to mimic the texture of breadcrumbs closely.
- For extra flavor, you can mix a small amount of the rosemary aioli into the patty mixture before cooking.
- Cooking the patties in butter not only adds flavor but also helps to achieve a golden and crispy exterior.

Spicy Beef Liver Patties with Chipotle Aioli

Prep Time: 20 minutes
Cook Time: 10 minutes
Total Time: 30 minutes
Servings: 4

Ingredients:

For the Patties:

- 1 lb beef liver, cleaned and finely minced
- 1 large egg
- 1/2 cup finely ground almond flour
- 1 medium onion, finely diced
- 2 cloves garlic, minced
- 1 teaspoon cumin
- 1/2 teaspoon smoked paprika
- 1/4 teaspoon cayenne pepper (adjust to taste)
- Salt and freshly ground black pepper, to taste
- 2 tablespoons olive oil, for frying

For the Chipotle Aioli:

- 1/2 cup mayonnaise

- 1 chipotle pepper in adobo sauce, minced
- 1 teaspoon adobo sauce (from the can of chipotle peppers)
- 1 clove garlic, minced
- 1 tablespoon lime juice
- Salt to taste

Instructions:

1. **Prepare the Patties:** In a large mixing bowl, combine minced beef liver, egg, almond flour, onion, garlic, cumin, smoked paprika, cayenne pepper, salt, and black pepper. Mix until all ingredients are well incorporated.

2. **Form Patties:** Shape the mixture into 8 small or 4 large patties, depending on your preference.

3. **Cook Patties:** Heat olive oil in a skillet over medium heat. Add the patties and cook for about 4-5 minutes on each side, until fully cooked and golden brown on the outside.

4. **Make the Chipotle Aioli:** While the patties are cooking, prepare the aioli by combining mayonnaise, minced chipotle pepper, adobo sauce,

minced garlic, lime juice, and salt in a small bowl. Stir until smooth.

5. **Serve:** Serve the beef liver patties hot, topped with or alongside the chipotle aioli for dipping.

Nutritional Information (per serving):

- Calories: 420
- Protein: 27g
- Fat: 32g
- Carbohydrates: 9g
- Cholesterol: 300mg
- Sodium: 400mg

Chef's Tips:

- Cleaning the liver thoroughly and removing any veins will ensure a smoother texture for the patties.
- The chipotle aioli can be adjusted for spiciness by adding more or less chipotle pepper and adobo sauce.
- Serve with lime wedges for an extra splash of citrus that complements the smoky, spicy flavors of the aioli.

Mediterranean Beef Liver Patties with Lemon Herb Aioli

Prep Time: 25 minutes
Cook Time: 10 minutes
Total Time: 35 minutes
Servings: 4

Ingredients:

For the Patties:

- 1 lb beef liver, finely minced

- 1/2 cup breadcrumbs (use pork rinds for a carnivore diet alternative)

- 2 large eggs, beaten

- 1/4 cup fresh parsley, finely chopped

- 1/4 cup fresh mint, finely chopped

- 2 cloves garlic, minced

- 1 small red onion, finely chopped

- Zest of 1 lemon

- Salt and freshly ground black pepper, to taste

- 2 tablespoons ghee or clarified butter, for frying

For the Lemon Herb Aioli:

- 1/2 cup mayonnaise
- 1 tablespoon fresh lemon juice
- 1 teaspoon lemon zest
- 1 tablespoon fresh parsley, finely chopped
- 1 clove garlic, minced
- Salt and pepper, to taste

Instructions:

1. **Prepare the Patties:** In a bowl, combine the minced beef liver, breadcrumbs (or pork rind crumbs), beaten eggs, parsley, mint, garlic, red onion, and lemon zest. Season with salt and pepper, and mix until well combined.

2. **Form Patties:** Shape the mixture into 8 small patties.

3. **Cook Patties:** Heat ghee in a skillet over medium heat. Fry the patties for about 5 minutes on each side, or until they are cooked through and have a golden-brown crust.

4. **Make the Lemon Herb Aioli:** In a small bowl, mix together mayonnaise, lemon juice, lemon zest,

parsley, and minced garlic. Season with salt and pepper to taste.

5. **Serve:** Arrange the beef liver patties on a platter and serve with the lemon herb aioli on the side for dipping.

   Nutritional Information (per serving):

- Calories: 435

- Protein: 28g

- Fat: 32g

- Carbohydrates: 10g (less if using pork rinds)

- Cholesterol: 345mg

Chicken Caesar Salad - A carnivore twist on a classic, using homemade anchovy dressing.

Classic Chicken Caesar Salad with Anchovy Dressing

Prep Time: 15 minutes
Cook Time: 20 minutes
Total Time: 35 minutes
Servings: 4

Ingredients:

For the Salad:

- 2 lbs chicken breast, grilled and sliced
- 4 cups Romaine lettuce, chopped (for a strict carnivore diet, substitute with additional protein options like hard-boiled eggs or extra chicken)
- 1/2 cup Parmesan cheese, shaved
- Optional for garnish: extra Parmesan shavings

For the Anchovy Dressing:

- 6 anchovy fillets, minced
- 1 clove garlic, minced
- 2 egg yolks

- 1 tablespoon lemon juice
- 1 teaspoon Dijon mustard
- 3/4 cup olive oil
- Salt and pepper, to taste

Instructions:

1. **Prepare the Dressing:** In a blender or food processor, combine minced anchovies, garlic, egg yolks, lemon juice, and Dijon mustard. Blend until smooth. With the blender running, slowly add the olive oil until the dressing is thick and emulsified. Season with salt and pepper to taste.

2. **Assemble the Salad:** In a large bowl, toss the chopped Romaine lettuce (or your chosen substitute) with a generous amount of the anchovy dressing until well coated.

3. **Add Chicken and Cheese:** Arrange the sliced grilled chicken on top of the dressed lettuce. Sprinkle with shaved Parmesan cheese.

4. **Serve:** Divide the salad among plates, garnish with extra Parmesan shavings if desired, and serve immediately.

Nutritional Information (per serving):

- Calories: 590
- Protein: 55g
- Fat: 37g
- Carbohydrates: 4g
- Cholesterol: 245mg
- Sodium: 620mg

Chef's Tips:

- For the best flavor, grill the chicken breast with a simple seasoning of salt and pepper to complement the rich dressing.
- Ensure the egg yolks and lemon juice are at room temperature before making the dressing to help them emulsify better.
- The dressing can be made ahead and stored in the refrigerator for up to 2 days; just whisk it well before using.

Grilled Chicken Caesar with Crispy Bacon Bits

Prep Time: 20 minutes
Cook Time: 20 minutes
Total Time: 40 minutes
Servings: 4

Ingredients:

For the Salad:

- 2 lbs chicken thighs, skin-on, grilled and sliced
- 4 cups Romaine lettuce, chopped (for a strict carnivore approach, consider adding more chicken or substituting with bacon bits)
- 1/2 cup Parmesan cheese, shaved
- 4 slices of bacon, cooked and crumbled

For the Anchovy Dressing:

- 4 anchovy fillets, minced
- 2 cloves garlic, minced
- 2 egg yolks
- 2 tablespoons lemon juice
- 1 tablespoon Worcestershire sauce (optional, for added umami)

- 3/4 cup olive oil

- Salt and pepper, to taste

Instructions:

1. **Prepare the Dressing:** In a blender, combine the anchovies, garlic, egg yolks, lemon juice, and Worcestershire sauce (if using). Blend until smooth. Gradually add the olive oil until the mixture is thick. Season with salt and pepper.

2. **Cook the Bacon:** In a skillet over medium heat, cook the bacon until crispy. Drain on paper towels and then crumble.

3. **Assemble the Salad:** Toss the chopped lettuce in a large bowl with enough dressing to coat. Add the sliced grilled chicken and bacon bits.

4. **Finish and Serve:** Top the salad with shaved Parmesan cheese. Serve immediately, offering additional dressing on the side if desired.

Nutritional Information (per serving):

- Calories: 650
- Protein: 60g
- Fat: 44g
- Carbohydrates: 3g
- Cholesterol: 270mg
- Sodium: 710mg

Chef's Tips:

- Grilling the chicken with the skin on helps keep it moist and adds extra flavor that pairs well with the salty anchovy dressing.
- For an extra touch of crunch, grill the Romaine lettuce cut-side down for a minute before chopping.
- If concerned about using raw egg yolks, look for pasteurized eggs or make a mayo-based dressing as an alternative.

Smoked Chicken Caesar Salad with Creamy Anchovy Dressing

Prep Time: 15 minutes (excluding smoking time)
Cook Time: 2 hours (for smoking chicken)
Total Time: 2 hours 15 minutes
Servings: 4

Ingredients:

For the Salad:

- 2 lbs whole chicken, smoked and shredded (skin removed for the salad)
- 4 cups Romaine lettuce, chopped (omit for a strict carnivore diet and double the chicken or substitute with cooked egg slices)
- 1/2 cup Parmesan cheese, shaved
- Lemon wedges for serving

For the Creamy Anchovy Dressing:

- 8 anchovy fillets, minced
- 1 clove garlic, minced
- 2 egg yolks
- 1 tablespoon lemon juice

- 1/2 cup mayonnaise
- Salt and pepper, to taste

Instructions:

1. **Smoke the Chicken:** Prepare your smoker for indirect cooking at 225°F (107°C). Smoke the whole chicken until the internal temperature reaches 165°F (74°C), about 2 hours. Let cool, then shred the meat, discarding the skin.

2. **Prepare the Dressing:** In a food processor, combine the minced anchovies, garlic, egg yolks, lemon juice, and mayonnaise. Process until smooth. Season with salt and pepper to taste.

3. **Assemble the Salad:** In a large bowl, toss the shredded smoked chicken with the creamy anchovy dressing until well coated. If using, gently mix in the chopped Romaine lettuce.

4. **Serve:** Plate the salad and top with shaved Parmesan cheese. Serve with lemon wedges on the side.

Nutritional Information (per serving):

- Calories: 680
- Protein: 58g
- Fat: 48g
- Carbohydrates: 3g (if omitting lettuce)
- Cholesterol: 295mg
- Sodium: 790mg

Chef's Tips:

- For optimal flavor, smoke the chicken with applewood or hickory chips to complement the creamy anchovy dressing.
- Shredding the chicken while it's still warm makes the process easier and ensures the meat absorbs more dressing flavor.
- The dressing can be prepared a day in advance and stored in the refrigerator to deepen the flavors.

Char-Grilled Chicken Caesar with Aged Parmesan Anchovy Dressing

Prep Time: 20 minutes
Cook Time: 15 minutes
Total Time: 35 minutes
Servings: 4

Ingredients:

For the Salad:

- 2 lbs chicken breast, boneless, skinless, grilled and sliced
- 4 cups Romaine lettuce, chopped (optional for carnivore diet adaptations)
- 1/2 cup aged Parmesan cheese, shaved
- Freshly ground black pepper, to taste

For the Aged Parmesan Anchovy Dressing:

- 6 anchovy fillets, minced
- 2 cloves garlic, minced
- 2 egg yolks
- 2 tablespoons lemon juice
- 3/4 cup olive oil

- 1/4 cup aged Parmesan cheese, finely grated
- Salt, to taste

Instructions:

1. **Grill the Chicken:** Preheat your grill to medium-high. Season the chicken breasts with salt and pepper, then grill for 6-7 minutes per side, or until fully cooked. Let rest for 5 minutes, then slice thinly.

2. **Prepare the Dressing:** In a blender, combine the anchovies, garlic, egg yolks, and lemon juice. Blend until smooth. With the blender running, slowly add the olive oil until the dressing thickens. Stir in the grated aged Parmesan cheese, and season with salt to taste.

3. **Assemble the Salad:** If including, toss the chopped Romaine lettuce in a large bowl with enough dressing to coat. Arrange the grilled chicken slices on top and sprinkle with shaved aged Parmesan cheese and freshly ground black pepper.

4. **Serve:** Divide the salad among plates, offering additional dressing on the side if desired.

Nutritional Information (per serving):

- Calories: 630
- Protein: 59g
- Fat: 40g
- Carbohydrates: 4g
- Cholesterol: 260mg
- Sodium: 820mg

Chef's Tips:

- Char-grilling the chicken adds a smoky depth of flavor that pairs well with the rich, umami-packed anchovy dressing.
- For the best texture and flavor, use high-quality aged Parmesan cheese both in the dressing and as a garnish.
- The dressing will thicken as it chills, so if made ahead, let it sit at room temperature for a few minutes before serving to loosen it up.

Classic Lamb Koftas with Yogurt Dip

Prep Time: 20 minutes
Cook Time: 10 minutes
Total Time: 30 minutes
Servings: 4

Ingredients:

For the Koftas:

- 1 lb ground lamb
- 2 cloves garlic, minced
- 1 small onion, finely grated
- 2 teaspoons cumin
- 1 teaspoon smoked paprika
- 1/2 teaspoon ground coriander
- 1/4 teaspoon cayenne pepper (adjust to taste)
- Salt and freshly ground black pepper, to taste
- Wooden or metal skewers (if using wooden skewers, soak in water for 30 minutes before using)

For the Yogurt Dip:

- 1 cup full-fat Greek yogurt
- 1 tablespoon lemon juice
- 1 tablespoon fresh mint, finely chopped
- Salt and pepper, to taste

Instructions:

1. **Prepare the Lamb Mixture:** In a large bowl, combine the ground lamb, minced garlic, grated onion, cumin, smoked paprika, ground coriander, cayenne pepper, salt, and black pepper. Mix until well combined.

2. **Form the Koftas:** Divide the mixture into 8 equal parts. Mold each part around a skewer into a long sausage shape. Press firmly to ensure the meat sticks to the skewer.

3. **Grill the Koftas:** Preheat your grill to medium-high heat. Grill the koftas for 4-5 minutes on each side, or until cooked through and slightly charred on the outside.

4. **Prepare the Yogurt Dip:** While the koftas are grilling, mix together Greek yogurt, lemon juice, chopped mint, salt, and pepper in a small bowl.

5. **Serve:** Serve the grilled lamb koftas hot with the yogurt dip on the side.

    Nutritional Information (per serving):

- Calories: 325

- Protein: 23g

- Fat: 24g

- Carbohydrates: 4g

- Cholesterol: 85mg

- Sodium: 200mg

    Chef's Tips:

- Ensure the grill is hot before adding the koftas to get a good sear and prevent sticking.

- Do not overmix the lamb mixture to keep the koftas tender.

- Resting the koftas for a few minutes after grilling allows the juices to redistribute, making them juicier.

Spicy Harissa Lamb Koftas

Prep Time: 30 minutes (including marinating time)
Cook Time: 10 minutes
Total Time: 40 minutes
Servings: 4

Ingredients:

For the Koftas:

- 1 lb ground lamb
- 2 tablespoons harissa paste
- 2 cloves garlic, minced
- 1 teaspoon ground cumin
- 1/2 teaspoon ground cinnamon
- 1/4 teaspoon ground allspice
- Salt and freshly ground black pepper, to taste
- Wooden or metal skewers

For the Harissa Yogurt Sauce:

- 1 cup full-fat Greek yogurt
- 1 tablespoon harissa paste

- 1 tablespoon olive oil
- Salt and pepper, to taste

Instructions:

1. **Marinate the Lamb:** In a bowl, combine ground lamb, harissa paste, minced garlic, cumin, cinnamon, allspice, salt, and pepper. Mix well and let marinate in the refrigerator for at least 20 minutes.

2. **Form the Koftas:** Divide the lamb mixture into 8 portions and form each around a skewer into a sausage shape.

3. **Grill the Koftas:** Preheat a grill or grill pan over medium-high heat. Grill the koftas for about 5 minutes on each side, until nicely charred and cooked through.

4. **Prepare the Harissa Yogurt Sauce:** Mix Greek yogurt, harissa paste, and olive oil in a bowl. Season with salt and pepper to taste.

5. **Serve:** Place the grilled koftas on a platter and serve with the harissa yogurt sauce on the side.

Nutritional Information (per serving):

- Calories: 360
- Protein: 24g
- Fat: 26g
- Carbohydrates: 6g
- Cholesterol: 90mg
- Sodium: 250mg

Chef's Tips:

- Adjust the amount of harissa paste according to your spice preference. Harissa can vary in heat.
- Letting the lamb marinate not only infuses it with flavor but also tenderizes the meat, resulting in juicier koftas.
- If using wooden skewers, soaking them in water prevents them from burning during grilling.

Mint and Garlic Lamb Koftas

Prep Time: 15 minutes
Cook Time: 10 minutes
Total Time: 25 minutes
Servings: 4

Ingredients:

For the Koftas:

- 1 lb ground lamb
- 1/4 cup fresh mint, finely chopped
- 3 cloves garlic, minced
- 1 small onion, finely grated
- 1 teaspoon ground cumin
- 1/2 teaspoon paprika
- 1/4 teaspoon cayenne pepper
- Salt and freshly ground black pepper, to taste
- Wooden or metal skewers

Instructions:

1. **Prepare the Kofta Mixture:** In a large mixing bowl, combine the ground lamb, chopped mint, minced garlic, grated onion, cumin, paprika, cayenne pepper, salt, and black pepper. Mix well until all ingredients are evenly distributed.

2. **Form the Koftas:** Divide the lamb mixture into 8 equal parts. Shape each portion around a skewer, forming a long, sausage-like shape. Make sure the meat is evenly distributed along the skewer.

3. **Grill the Koftas:** Preheat your grill or grill pan to medium-high heat. Place the koftas on the grill and cook for about 5 minutes on each side, turning occasionally, until they are well-browned and cooked through.

4. **Serve:** Remove the koftas from the grill and allow them to rest for a few minutes before serving. They can be served with a side of tzatziki sauce or a simple salad for a complete meal.

Nutritional Information (per serving):

- Calories: 330
- Protein: 22g
- Fat: 25g

- Carbohydrates: 3g
- Cholesterol: 90mg
- Sodium: 75mg

Chef's Tips:

- Fresh mint is key to the flavor profile of these koftas; however, a combination of mint and parsley can also be used for a different twist.
- Ensuring the grill is properly heated before adding the koftas will prevent sticking and ensure a good sear.
- Resting the koftas after grilling helps to redistribute the juices, keeping them moist and flavorful.

Herb-Infused Lamb Koftas with Cucumber Yogurt Sauce

Prep Time: 20 minutes (including marinating time)
Cook Time: 10 minutes
Total Time: 30 minutes
Servings: 4

Ingredients:

For the Koftas:

- 1 lb ground lamb
- 2 tablespoons fresh parsley, finely chopped
- 2 tablespoons fresh cilantro, finely chopped
- 1 teaspoon dried oregano
- 2 cloves garlic, minced
- 1/2 teaspoon ground coriander
- 1/4 teaspoon ground cinnamon
- Salt and freshly ground black pepper, to taste
- Wooden or metal skewers

For the Cucumber Yogurt Sauce:

- 1 cup Greek yogurt

- 1/2 cucumber, grated and excess water squeezed out
- 2 tablespoons lemon juice
- 1 tablespoon olive oil
- 1 clove garlic, minced
- Salt and pepper, to taste

Instructions:

1. **Marinate the Lamb:** In a bowl, mix together the ground lamb, parsley, cilantro, oregano, minced garlic, coriander, cinnamon, salt, and pepper. Let the mixture marinate in the refrigerator for at least 15 minutes.

2. **Prepare the Sauce:** While the lamb is marinating, prepare the cucumber yogurt sauce by combining Greek yogurt, grated cucumber, lemon juice, olive oil, minced garlic, salt, and pepper in a bowl. Mix well and refrigerate until ready to serve.

3. **Form and Cook the Koftas:** Preheat your grill to medium-high heat. Divide the lamb mixture into 8 portions and shape each around a skewer. Grill the koftas for about 5 minutes on each side, or until cooked through and slightly charred.

4. **Serve:** Serve the koftas hot with the cucumber yogurt sauce on the side.

Nutritional Information (per serving):

- Calories: 360
- Protein: 23g
- Fat: 27g
- Carbohydrates: 5g
- Cholesterol: 85mg
- Sodium: 80mg

Chef's Tips:

- Draining the grated cucumber before adding it to the yogurt helps prevent the sauce from becoming too watery.
- For an extra flavor boost, let the lamb mixture marinate overnight in the refrigerator.
- If using wooden skewers, soaking them in water for at least 30 minutes before grilling will prevent them from burning.

Dinner Recipes

Ribeye with Bone Marrow Butter - A luxurious main course.

Classic Ribeye with Bone Marrow Butter

Prep Time: 15 minutes (plus time for marrow butter to set)
Cook Time: 10 minutes
Total Time: 25 minutes (excluding butter setting time)
Servings: 2

Ingredients:

For the Ribeye:

- 2 ribeye steaks (about 1 inch thick)
- Salt and freshly ground black pepper, to taste
- 2 tablespoons olive oil

For the Bone Marrow Butter:

- 4 ounces bone marrow, scooped from bones
- 1/2 cup unsalted butter, softened
- 1 clove garlic, minced

- 1 tablespoon fresh parsley, finely chopped
- Salt and freshly ground black pepper, to taste

Instructions:

1. **Prepare the Bone Marrow Butter:** In a small pan, gently cook the bone marrow over low heat until melted. Strain and let cool slightly. Mix the melted marrow with softened butter, minced garlic, parsley, salt, and pepper. Place the mixture on a piece of plastic wrap, roll into a log, and refrigerate until firm.

2. **Cook the Ribeye:** Season the ribeye steaks generously with salt and pepper. Heat olive oil in a heavy skillet over high heat until smoking. Add the steaks and cook for about 4-5 minutes on each side for medium-rare, or to your desired doneness. Let the steaks rest for 5 minutes after cooking.

3. **Serve:** Slice the bone marrow butter and place a piece on top of each hot steak, allowing it to melt over the meat.

4. **Enjoy:** Serve immediately, accompanied by your favorite side dishes.

Nutritional Information (per serving):

- Calories: 750
- Protein: 45g
- Fat: 65g
- Carbohydrates: 0g
- Cholesterol: 180mg
- Sodium: 120mg

Chef's Tips:

- Allowing the steak to rest before serving is crucial for retaining its juices and ensuring maximum flavor.
- For an extra depth of flavor, consider adding a splash of red wine to the skillet after removing the steaks, scraping up any browned bits for a simple pan sauce.
- The bone marrow butter can be made in advance and stored in the freezer. Slice off rounds as needed for a luxurious finish to steaks, vegetables, or even toast.

Herb-Crusted Ribeye with Roasted Garlic Bone Marrow Butter

Prep Time: 20 minutes (plus time for butter to set)
Cook Time: 15 minutes
Total Time: 35 minutes (excluding butter setting time)
Servings: 2

Ingredients:

For the Ribeye:

- 2 ribeye steaks (about 1.5 inches thick)
- 1 tablespoon fresh rosemary, finely chopped
- 1 tablespoon fresh thyme, finely chopped
- Salt and freshly ground black pepper, to taste
- 2 tablespoons olive oil

For the Roasted Garlic Bone Marrow Butter:

- 4 ounces bone marrow
- 1/2 head garlic, roasted and cloves squeezed out
- 1/2 cup unsalted butter, room temperature
- Salt and freshly ground black pepper, to taste

Instructions:

1. **Prepare the Roasted Garlic Bone Marrow Butter:** Roast the bone marrow in a preheated oven at 350°F (175°C) for 15 minutes. Let cool, then mix the marrow with the roasted garlic and softened butter in a bowl. Season with salt and pepper, form into a log using plastic wrap, and refrigerate until firm.

2. **Season the Ribeye:** Combine rosemary, thyme, salt, and pepper. Rub this herb mixture all over the ribeye steaks.

3. **Cook the Steaks:** Heat olive oil in a skillet over high heat. Once hot, add the steaks and cook for 6-7 minutes on each side for medium-rare, or adjust the time for your preferred doneness. Let the steaks rest for at least 5 minutes after cooking.

4. **Serve:** Top each steak with a slice of the roasted garlic bone marrow butter, allowing it to melt over the warm steak.

5. **Enjoy:** Serve the steaks immediately, basking in the luxurious flavors.

Nutritional Information (per serving):

- Calories: 800
- Protein: 48g
- Fat: 68g
- Carbohydrates: 2g
- Cholesterol: 190mg
- Sodium: 130mg

Chef's Tips:

- Roasting the garlic for the marrow butter adds a sweet, mellow depth that complements the richness of the marrow.

- Pressing the herb crust onto the steaks before cooking ensures a flavorful, aromatic crust.

- Allow the bone marrow butter to soften slightly before serving for easier

Pepper-Crusted Ribeye with Thyme Bone Marrow Butter

Prep

Time: 20 minutes (plus chilling time for butter)
Cook Time: 10 minutes
Total Time: 30 minutes
Servings: 2

Ingredients:

For the Ribeye:

- 2 ribeye steaks (about 1 inch thick each)
- 1 tablespoon coarse ground black pepper
- 1 teaspoon sea salt
- 2 tablespoons olive oil

For the Thyme Bone Marrow Butter:

- 4 ounces bone marrow, roasted and mashed
- 1/2 cup unsalted butter, softened
- 1 tablespoon fresh thyme leaves
- 1 clove garlic, minced
- Salt to taste

Instructions:

1. **Prepare the Thyme Bone Marrow Butter:** Combine the mashed bone marrow, softened butter, thyme leaves, minced garlic, and salt in a bowl. Mix until well blended. Place the mixture on a piece of plastic wrap, form into a log, and chill in the refrigerator until firm.

2. **Season the Ribeye:** Rub both sides of each ribeye steak with coarse ground black pepper and sea salt.

3. **Cook the Ribeye:** Heat olive oil in a heavy skillet over high heat. Once hot, add the ribeye steaks and cook for 5 minutes on one side, then flip and cook for another 4-5 minutes for medium-rare, or cook to your desired level of doneness.

4. **Serve:** Place the cooked ribeye steaks on plates. Slice the thyme bone marrow butter and place a piece on top of each steak, allowing it to melt over the meat.

5. **Enjoy:** Serve immediately, accompanied by your choice of side dishes.

Nutritional Information (per serving):

- Calories: 780
- Protein: 50g

- Fat: 65g
- Carbohydrates: 1g
- Cholesterol: 180mg
- Sodium: 600mg

    Chef's Tips:

- Allowing the steak to rest for 5 minutes before serving helps retain its juices, resulting in a more flavorful and tender steak.
- For an even crust of pepper, press the seasoning into the meat before cooking.
- The bone marrow butter can also be used to top vegetables or roasted potatoes, adding a rich, savory flavor.

Smoky Ribeye with Chipotle Bone Marrow Butter

Prep Time: 15 minutes (plus chilling time for butter)
Cook Time: 10 minutes
Total Time: 25 minutes
Servings: 2

Ingredients:

For the Ribeye:

- 2 ribeye steaks (about 1.5 inches thick each)
- 1 teaspoon smoked paprika
- Salt and freshly ground black pepper, to taste
- 2 tablespoons grapeseed oil or another high-smoke-point oil

For the Chipotle Bone Marrow Butter:

- 4 ounces bone marrow, roasted and mashed
- 1/2 cup unsalted butter, at room temperature
- 1 chipotle pepper in adobo sauce, finely chopped
- 1 teaspoon adobo sauce (from the chipotle peppers can)

- Salt to taste

Instructions:

1. **Prepare the Chipotle Bone Marrow Butter:** In a bowl, mix together the mashed bone marrow, butter, chopped chipotle pepper, adobo sauce, and salt until well combined. Transfer the mixture to plastic wrap, roll into a log shape, and refrigerate until firm.

2. **Season the Ribeye:** Season both sides of the ribeye steaks with smoked paprika, salt, and pepper.

3. **Cook the Ribeye:** Heat grapeseed oil in a skillet over high heat. Add the ribeye steaks and cook for about 5 minutes on one side, then flip and cook for another 4-5 minutes for medium-rare, or until desired doneness is reached.

4. **Serve:** Transfer the steaks to plates. Cut slices of the chipotle bone marrow butter and place on top of each hot steak, allowing the butter to melt and infuse the steak with its smoky, spicy flavors.

5. **Enjoy:** Serve the ribeye steaks immediately, savoring the rich and complex flavors.

Nutritional Information (per serving):

- Calories: 800
- Protein: 52g
- Fat: 68g
- Carbohydrates: 2g
- Cholesterol: 185mg
- Sodium: 610mg

Chef's Tips:

- For a more pronounced smoky flavor, consider adding a pinch of ground chipotle powder to the steak along with the smoked paprika.
- Ensure the steaks are at room temperature before cooking to promote even cooking and browning.
- The chipotle bone marrow butter adds a spicy kick that complements the richness of the ribeye.

Duck Breast with Red Wine Reduction - Elegant, with a focus on technique.

Seared Duck Breast with Classic Red Wine Reduction

Prep	**Time:**	10	minutes
Cook	**Time:**	25	minutes
Total	**Time:**	35	minutes

Servings: 2

Ingredients:

For the Duck:

- 2 duck breasts, skin on
- Salt and freshly ground black pepper, to taste

For the Red Wine Reduction:

- 1 cup red wine (Pinot Noir or Merlot works well)
- 2 tablespoons shallots, finely chopped
- 1 clove garlic, minced
- 1 sprig fresh thyme
- 1/2 cup beef or duck stock
- Salt and freshly ground black pepper, to taste

Instructions:

1. **Prepare the Duck Breasts:** Score the skin of the duck breasts in a crosshatch pattern, being careful not to cut into the meat. Season both sides with salt and pepper.

2. **Cook the Duck:** Preheat a skillet over medium heat. Place the duck breasts skin-side down and cook for 8-10 minutes, or until the skin is golden and crisp. Flip and cook on the flesh side for another 5-7 minutes for medium-rare. Remove from the skillet and let rest for 5 minutes.

3. **Make the Red Wine Reduction:** In the same skillet, sauté shallots and garlic until softened. Add the red wine and thyme, scraping up any browned bits from the bottom of the skillet. Simmer until reduced by half, then add the stock. Continue to simmer until the sauce has thickened. Season with salt and pepper. Strain the sauce for a smoother texture if desired.

4. **Serve:** Slice the duck breasts and serve with the red wine reduction drizzled over the top.

Nutritional Information (per serving):

- Calories: 480
- Protein: 45g
- Fat: 22g
- Carbohydrates: 8g
- Cholesterol: 195mg
- Sodium: 620mg

Chef's Tips:

- Scoring the duck skin helps render the fat and achieve a crispy finish.
- Letting the duck rest before slicing ensures that the juices redistribute, making the meat more tender and flavorful.
- The red wine reduction can be prepared in advance and gently reheated, adding a touch of butter for extra richness just before serving.

Duck Breast with Berry and Red Wine Jus

Prep Time: 15 minutes
Cook Time: 20 minutes
Total Time: 35 minutes
Servings: 2

Ingredients:

For the Duck:

- 2 duck breasts, skin on
- Salt and freshly ground black pepper, to taste

For the Berry and Red Wine Jus:

- 3/4 cup red wine (Cabernet Sauvignon works well)
- 1/4 cup mixed berries (raspberries, blackberries, or blueberries)
- 2 tablespoons balsamic vinegar
- 1 tablespoon honey
- 1 sprig of rosemary
- Salt and freshly ground black pepper, to taste

Instructions:

1. **Prepare the Duck Breasts:** Score the skin of the duck breasts without cutting into the meat. Season with salt and pepper.

2. **Cook the Duck:** Place the duck breasts skin-side down in a cold skillet. Turn the heat to medium and cook until the skin is crisp, about 8-10 minutes. Flip and cook on the flesh side for 5-7 minutes for medium-rare. Remove and let rest.

3. **Make the Berry and Red Wine Jus:** In the same skillet, add the red wine, mixed berries, balsamic vinegar, honey, and rosemary. Simmer until the sauce is reduced by half and thickened, stirring occasionally. Season with salt and pepper.

4. **Serve:** Slice the rested duck breasts and serve with the berry and red wine jus spooned over the top.

Nutritional Information (per serving):

- Calories: 510
- Protein: 46g
- Fat: 24g
- Carbohydrates: 15g

- Cholesterol: 200mg
- Sodium: 630mg

Chef's Tips:

- Starting the duck in a cold skillet helps render the fat more effectively for a crispier skin.
- The addition of berries to the red wine jus introduces a subtle sweetness and tartness that complements the richness of the duck.
- For a smoother sauce, you can strain the jus before serving to remove the berry solids and rosemary sprig.

Duck Breast with Shallot Red Wine Sauce

Prep Time: 15 minutes
Cook Time: 25 minutes
Total Time: 40 minutes
Servings: 2

Ingredients:

For the Duck:

- 2 duck breasts, skin scored
- Salt and freshly ground black pepper, to taste

For the Shallot Red Wine Sauce:

- 1 cup good quality red wine (such as Shiraz or Bordeaux)
- 1/4 cup finely diced shallots
- 2 tablespoons unsalted butter
- 1 teaspoon sugar
- 1/2 cup chicken or duck stock
- Salt and freshly ground black pepper, to taste
- A few sprigs of thyme

Instructions:

1. **Season the Duck:** Season the duck breasts generously with salt and pepper.

2. **Cook the Duck:** Heat a skillet over medium-low heat. Place the duck breasts skin-side down and cook for about 10 minutes, until the skin is crispy. Turn over and cook for another 5-8 minutes for medium-rare. Remove from the skillet and let rest.

3. **Prepare the Sauce:** In the same skillet, add the shallots and cook until softened, about 2-3 minutes. Pour in the red wine, add sugar, and increase the heat to bring to a simmer. Reduce the wine by half, then add the stock and thyme. Simmer until the sauce thickens slightly. Whisk in the butter, season with salt and pepper, and strain the sauce.

4. **Serve:** Slice the duck breast and serve with the shallot red wine sauce drizzled over the top.

Nutritional Information (per serving):

- Calories: 540
- Protein: 48g
- Fat: 28g
- Carbohydrates: 12g

- Cholesterol: 220mg
- Sodium: 350mg

Chef's Tips:

- Scoring the skin of the duck breast helps render the fat for a crispier finish.
- Resting the duck before slicing ensures juiciness and flavor.
- The addition of sugar to the sauce balances the acidity of the wine and enhances the depth of flavor.

Duck Breast with Fig and Red Wine Reduction

Prep Time: 20 minutes
Cook Time: 30 minutes
Total Time: 50 minutes
Servings: 2

Ingredients:

For the Duck:

- 2 duck breasts, skin scored
- Salt and freshly ground black pepper, to taste

For the Fig and Red Wine Reduction:

- 1 cup red wine (a fruity variety works well)
- 1/2 cup fresh figs, quartered
- 2 tablespoons honey
- 1 clove garlic, minced
- 1 sprig rosemary
- 1/2 cup beef or duck stock
- Salt and freshly ground black pepper, to taste

Instructions:

1. **Prepare the Duck:** Season the duck breasts with salt and pepper.

2. **Cook the Duck:** Place the duck breasts skin-side down in a cold skillet. Turn the heat to medium and cook until the fat renders and the skin is golden brown, about 10 minutes. Flip the breasts and cook to your desired doneness, about 5-7 minutes for medium-rare. Remove and let rest.

3. **Make the Reduction:** In the same skillet, combine the red wine, figs, honey, garlic, and rosemary. Bring to a simmer and cook until the wine is reduced by half. Add the stock and continue to simmer until the sauce thickens. Season with salt and pepper.

4. **Serve:** Slice the duck and arrange on plates. Spoon the fig and red wine reduction over the duck and serve immediately.

Nutritional Information (per serving):

- Calories: 560
- Protein: 49g
- Fat: 27g
- Carbohydrates: 23g
- Cholesterol: 225mg
- Sodium: 360mg

Chef's Tips:

- Fresh figs add a natural sweetness to the sauce that complements the duck's richness.
- Starting the duck in a cold pan helps render the fat more effectively, ensuring crispy skin.
- Allowing the sauce to reduce and thicken not only intensifies the flavor but also creates a luxurious texture perfect for drizzling.

Slow-Cooked Pork Shoulder - A simple, versatile recipe that can feed you for days.

Classic Slow-Cooked Pork Shoulder with Herbs

Prep Time: 15 minutes
Cook Time: 8 hours
Total Time: 8 hours 15 minutes
Servings: 8

Ingredients:

- 5 lb pork shoulder
- 2 tablespoons sea salt
- 1 tablespoon black pepper
- 1 tablespoon dried rosemary
- 1 tablespoon dried thyme
- 4 cloves garlic, minced
- 2 tablespoons olive oil

Instructions:

1. **Prepare the Pork:** Pat the pork shoulder dry with paper towels. In a small bowl, mix together the sea salt, black pepper, dried rosemary, dried thyme, and minced garlic.

2. **Season:** Rub the olive oil all over the pork shoulder, then evenly coat it with the herb and garlic mixture.

3. **Slow Cook:** Place the seasoned pork shoulder in a slow cooker. Cover and set to cook on low for 8 hours or until the pork is very tender and easily shreds with a fork.

4. **Rest and Serve:** Once cooked, let the pork shoulder rest for 10-15 minutes before shredding. Serve warm.

Nutritional Information (per serving):

- Calories: 510
- Protein: 65g
- Fat: 25g
- Carbohydrates: 1g
- Cholesterol: 180mg
- Sodium: 900mg

Chef's Tips:

- Allowing the pork to rest before shredding locks in moisture, resulting in a juicier dish.

- The pork can be shredded and used in various meals throughout the week, from salads to tacos or as a hearty main dish.

- For added flavor, consider adding a cup of chicken or vegetable broth to the slow cooker before cooking.

Spicy Slow-Cooked Pork Shoulder with Smoked Paprika

Prep Time: 15 minutes
Cook Time: 8 hours
Total Time: 8 hours 15 minutes
Servings: 8

Ingredients:

- 5 lb pork shoulder
- 2 tablespoons sea salt
- 1 tablespoon smoked paprika
- 1 teaspoon cayenne pepper (adjust based on heat preference)
- 1 tablespoon garlic powder
- 1 tablespoon onion powder
- 2 tablespoons olive oil

Instructions:

1. **Prepare the Pork:** Dry the pork shoulder with paper towels. Combine the sea salt, smoked paprika, cayenne pepper, garlic powder, and onion powder in a bowl.

2. **Season:** Rub the pork shoulder with olive oil, then coat it thoroughly with the spice mix.

3. **Slow Cook:** Transfer the pork shoulder to a slow cooker. Cover and cook on low for 8 hours, or until the meat is tender and falls apart easily.

4. **Rest and Serve:** Let the pork shoulder rest for a few minutes after cooking, then shred it with two forks. Serve as desired, enjoying the spicy flavors.

Nutritional Information (per serving):

- Calories: 520
- Protein: 66g
- Fat: 26g
- Carbohydrates: 2g
- Cholesterol: 185mg
- Sodium: 920mg

Chef's Tips:

- For a smokier flavor, you can add a teaspoon of liquid smoke to the rub.
- This recipe is perfect for meal prep, as the shredded pork can be used in a variety of dishes throughout the week.
- Serving suggestion: The spicy shredded pork pairs excellently with low-carb cauliflower rice or wrapped in lettuce leaves for a light yet satisfying meal.

Garlic and Lemon Slow-Cooked Pork Shoulder

Prep Time: 20 minutes
Cook Time: 8 to 10 hours
Total Time: 8 hours 20 minutes to 10 hours 20 minutes
Servings: 8

Ingredients:

- 5 lb pork shoulder
- 1/4 cup olive oil
- 6 cloves garlic, minced
- Zest of 2 lemons
- 2 tablespoons fresh rosemary, chopped
- 2 tablespoons sea salt
- 1 tablespoon freshly ground black pepper

Instructions:

1. **Prepare the Pork:** Rinse the pork shoulder and pat it dry with paper towels.
2. **Make the Marinade:** In a bowl, mix together olive oil, minced garlic, lemon zest, chopped rosemary, sea salt, and black pepper to create a paste.

3. **Marinate:** Rub the paste all over the pork shoulder, ensuring it is evenly coated. If time allows, let the pork marinate in the refrigerator for a few hours or overnight to enhance the flavors.

4. **Slow Cook:** Place the marinated pork shoulder in a slow cooker. Cover and set it to cook on low for 8 to 10 hours, or until the pork is tender and falls apart easily with a fork.

5. **Serve:** Once cooked, let the pork rest for 10-15 minutes before shredding. Serve the shredded pork with some of the cooking juices drizzled over the top.

Nutritional Information (per serving):

- Calories: 520
- Protein: 67g
- Fat: 28g
- Carbohydrates: 1g
- Cholesterol: 190mg
- Sodium: 1,750mg

Chef's Tips:

- The lemon zest adds a fresh, tangy flavor to the pork, cutting through the richness of the meat.

- For a crispy finish, after shredding, spread the pork on a baking sheet and broil for a few minutes until the edges are crispy.

- Leftovers can be used in a variety of ways, such as in sandwiches, salads, or as a protein addition to breakfast dishes.

Slow-Cooked Pork Shoulder with Apple Cider Vinegar

Prep Time: 15 minutes
Cook Time: 8 hours
Total Time: 8 hours 15 minutes
Servings: 8

Ingredients:

- 5 lb pork shoulder
- 1/4 cup apple cider vinegar
- 1/4 cup water
- 2 tablespoons brown sugar (omit for a strict carnivore diet, or substitute with a carnivore diet-approved sweetener)
- 1 tablespoon smoked paprika
- 2 teaspoons garlic powder
- 2 teaspoons onion powder
- 2 teaspoons sea salt
- 1 teaspoon freshly ground black pepper

Instructions:

1. **Prepare the Pork:** Rinse the pork shoulder and pat it dry. Mix the smoked paprika, garlic powder, onion powder, sea salt, and black pepper in a small bowl.

2. **Season:** Rub the spice mix all over the pork shoulder. Place the pork in a slow cooker.

3. **Mix the Liquid:** In a separate bowl, whisk together apple cider vinegar, water, and brown sugar (if using). Pour the mixture over the pork in the slow cooker.

4. **Cook:** Cover and cook on low for 8 hours, or until the pork is very tender.

5. **Finish and Serve:** Remove the pork from the slow cooker and let it rest for a few minutes before shredding with two forks. Serve hot with your choice of sides or use it in various dishes throughout the week.

Nutritional Information (per serving):

- Calories: 510
- Protein: 68g
- Fat: 25g
- Carbohydrates: 2g (without brown sugar)
- Cholesterol: 185mg
- Sodium: 660mg

Chef's Tips:

- The apple cider vinegar adds a tangy flavor that complements the richness of the pork.
- For those on a strict carnivore diet, the addition of brown sugar can be skipped or replaced with a suitable alternative that adheres to dietary restrictions.
- Shredding the pork and then briefly broiling it can add a delicious crispy texture to the edges.

Snacks Recipes

Spiced Crispy Chicken Skins

Prep Time: 10 minutes
Cook Time: 40 minutes
Total Time: 50 minutes
Servings: 4

Ingredients:

- Skin from 4 chicken thighs
- 1 teaspoon sea salt
- 1/2 teaspoon ground black pepper
- 1/2 teaspoon smoked paprika (optional for a carnivore diet, but adds flavor)
- 1/4 teaspoon garlic powder (optional for a carnivore diet, but adds flavor)

Instructions:

1. Prepare the Chicken Skins: Preheat your oven to 375°F (190°C). Remove any excess fat from the chicken skins and lay them flat on a baking sheet lined with parchment paper.

2. Season: Sprinkle the sea salt, ground black pepper, smoked paprika, and garlic powder evenly over the chicken skins.

3. Bake: Place another piece of parchment paper on top of the chicken skins, then place another baking sheet on top to keep them flat. Bake in the preheated oven for 35-40 minutes, or until crispy and golden brown.

4. Cool and Serve: Remove the chicken skins from the oven and let them cool on a wire rack to maintain crispiness. Serve as a crunchy, chip-like snack.

Nutritional Information (per serving):

- Calories: 150
- Protein: 14g
- Fat: 10g
- Carbohydrates: 0g
- Cholesterol: 40mg
- Sodium: 600mg

Chef's Tips:

- Keeping a second baking sheet on top of the chicken skins during baking helps them stay flat and cook evenly.

- Letting the chicken skins cool on a wire rack ensures they stay crispy.

- Adjust the seasoning according to your taste preferences or dietary needs.

Simple Salted Crispy Chicken Skins

Prep Time: 5 minutes
Cook Time: 35 minutes
Total Time: 40 minutes
Servings: 4

Ingredients:

- Skin from 4 chicken thighs
- 1 teaspoon coarse sea salt

Instructions:

1. Preheat the Oven: Preheat your oven to 375°F (190°C). Prepare a baking sheet by lining it with parchment paper.

2. Prepare the Skins: Trim any excess fat from the chicken skins and lay them out flat on the prepared baking sheet.

3. Season: Evenly sprinkle the coarse sea salt over the chicken skins.

4. Bake: Place the chicken skins in the oven and bake for 30-35 minutes, or until they are crispy and golden. There's no need to cover them with another baking sheet unless you prefer them extra flat.

5. Cool and Serve: Once done, transfer the crispy skins to a wire rack to cool. This ensures they stay crunchy.

Nutritional Information (per serving):

- Calories: 140
- Protein: 13g
- Fat: 9g
- Carbohydrates: 0g
- Cholesterol: 35mg
- Sodium: 590mg

Chef's Tips:

- For extra crispiness, consider increasing the oven temperature to 400°F (205°C) and reducing the cooking time slightly. Keep a close eye on them to prevent burning.

- These crispy skins can be stored in an airtight container for a few days, but they're best enjoyed fresh from the oven.

- Experiment with different types of salt, such as Himalayan pink salt or flaked sea salt, for varying textures and flavors.

Herbed Crispy Chicken Skins

Prep Time: 10 minutes
Cook Time: 40 minutes
Total Time: 50 minutes
Servings: 4

Ingredients:

- Skin from 4 chicken breasts
- 1 teaspoon fine sea salt
- 1/2 teaspoon cracked black pepper
- 1/2 teaspoon dried rosemary, finely crushed
- 1/2 teaspoon dried thyme
- Olive oil spray (optional, for a slight crisp)

Instructions:

1. **Preheat Oven:** Set your oven to 375°F (190°C). Line a baking sheet with parchment paper for easy cleanup.

2. **Prepare Chicken Skins:** Trim any excess fat from the chicken skins. Pat them dry with paper towels to ensure they get extra crispy.

3. **Season:** Lay the skins flat on the prepared baking sheet. Lightly spray with olive oil (if using), then evenly sprinkle sea salt, black pepper, rosemary, and thyme over them.

4. **Bake:** To keep the skins flat while baking, cover them with another piece of parchment paper, then place a second baking sheet on top. Bake in the preheated oven for 35-40 minutes, or until they reach desired crispiness.

5. **Serve:** Allow the chicken skins to cool on a wire rack to maintain their crisp texture. Enjoy as a savory, herby snack.

Nutritional Information (per serving):

- Calories: 135
- Protein: 15g
- Fat: 8g
- Carbohydrates: 0g
- Cholesterol: 45mg
- Sodium: 630mg

Chef's Tips:

- Drying the chicken skins thoroughly before baking is crucial for achieving the ultimate crisp.
- The herbs can be adjusted according to preference; mixing different combinations can create unique flavors.
- These crispy skins are best enjoyed immediately but can be reheated in the oven to restore crispness.

Parmesan Crusted Crispy Chicken Skins

Prep Time: 5 minutes
Cook Time: 40 minutes
Total Time: 45 minutes
Servings: 4

Ingredients:

- Skin from 4 chicken drumsticks
- 1 teaspoon kosher salt
- 1/2 teaspoon ground black pepper
- 1/4 cup grated Parmesan cheese

Instructions:

1. **Oven Preparation:** Heat your oven to 375°F (190°C) and line a baking tray with parchment paper.

2. **Skin Preparation:** Remove any excess fat from the chicken skins and lay them flat on the baking tray.

3. **Season:** Sprinkle the skins with kosher salt and ground black pepper, then gently press the grated Parmesan cheese onto each skin.

4. **Bake:** Place the chicken skins in the oven without covering them. Bake for about 40 minutes, or until they are crispy and the cheese has turned golden brown.

5. **Cooling:** Transfer the crispy skins to a wire rack to cool, ensuring they keep their crunch.

6. **Enjoy:** Serve these cheesy, crispy delights as a high-protein, low-carb snack.

Nutritional Information (per serving):

- Calories: 160
- Protein: 17g
- Fat: 9g
- Carbohydrates: 1g
- Cholesterol: 50mg
- Sodium: 720mg

Chef's Tips:

- The Parmesan cheese not only adds flavor but also aids in achieving a golden, crispy crust.
- Be careful to spread the skins out so they don't overlap on the baking tray, ensuring even cooking and crispiness.
- These can be served as a standalone snack or broken up as a crunchy salad topping for extra texture.

Beef Jerky - Homemade, no additives.

Simple Salt & Pepper Crispy Beef Jerky

Prep Time: 1 hour (for slicing and marinating)
Cook Time: 4 hours
Total Time: 5 hours
Servings: 6

Ingredients:

- 2 lbs lean beef (top round or flank steak works well)
- 2 tablespoons coarse sea salt
- 1 tablespoon cracked black pepper

Instructions:

1. **Prepare the Beef:** Freeze the beef for about 30 minutes to firm it up, making it easier to slice. Cut the beef against the grain into thin strips, approximately 1/8-inch thick.

2. **Season:** Lay the beef strips in a single layer on a baking sheet. Evenly sprinkle the sea salt and cracked black pepper on both sides of the beef strips. Let them marinate in the refrigerator for about 30 minutes.

3. **Oven Drying:** Preheat your oven to 175°F (80°C). Place the beef strips on a wire rack over a baking sheet to allow airflow. Bake for about 4 hours, or until the jerky is dry and firm, yet still pliable.

4. **Cool and Store:** Allow the jerky to cool completely before transferring it to an airtight container for storage.

Nutritional Information (per serving):

- Calories: 240
- Protein: 38g
- Fat: 8g
- Carbohydrates: 0g
- Cholesterol: 100mg
- Sodium: 2,330mg

Chef's Tips:

- Slicing the beef thinly and evenly ensures that the jerky dries uniformly.
- The longer the beef marinates with the salt and pepper, the more intense the flavors will be.

- Store the jerky in a cool, dry place to extend its shelf life.

Smoky Garlic Crispy Beef Jerky

Prep Time: 2 hours (for marinating)
Cook Time: 4 hours
Total Time: 6 hours
Servings: 6

Ingredients:

- 2 lbs lean beef (eye of round is a great choice)
- 2 tablespoons smoked sea salt
- 1 tablespoon garlic powder
- 1 teaspoon onion powder
- 1/2 teaspoon ground black pepper

Instructions:

1. **Prepare the Beef:** Partially freeze the beef for easier slicing. Cut the meat against the grain into thin, even strips, no thicker than 1/8 inch.

2. **Marinate:** Combine the smoked sea salt, garlic powder, onion powder, and black pepper in a bowl. Rub this mixture all over the beef strips. Place the seasoned beef in a covered container and refrigerate for at least 2 hours to marinate.

3. **Dry the Beef:** Preheat your oven to 175°F (80°C). Arrange the beef strips on a wire rack set over a baking sheet to catch drips. Ensure none of the strips are touching for proper airflow.

4. **Bake:** Dry the beef in the oven for approximately 4 hours, or until the jerky is dry but still pliable.

5. **Cool and Enjoy:** Let the jerky cool to room temperature before serving. Store leftovers in an airtight container.

Nutritional Information (per serving):

- Calories: 245
- Protein: 39g
- Fat: 7g
- Carbohydrates: 1g
- Cholesterol: 95mg
- Sodium: 2,360mg

Chef's Tips:

- Using smoked sea salt adds a natural smoky flavor without the need for a smoker.

- Ensure your oven is at the correct low temperature to dry the jerky without cooking it.

- Jerky can be stored in an airtight container for several weeks, but it's so delicious, it probably won't last that long!

Classic Teriyaki Beef Jerky

Prep Time: 1 hour (for slicing and marinating)
Cook Time: 4 hours
Total Time: 5 hours
Servings: 6

Ingredients:

- 2 lbs lean beef (sirloin or brisket works well)
- 1/4 cup soy sauce (use a natural, no-additive brand for a healthier option)
- 2 tablespoons apple cider vinegar
- 1 tablespoon honey (optional for a hint of sweetness, omit for strict carnivore diet)
- 1 teaspoon ground ginger
- 2 cloves garlic, minced
- 1/2 teaspoon black pepper

Instructions:

1. **Prepare the Beef:** Partially freeze the beef for easier slicing. Slice against the grain into thin strips, about 1/8-inch thick.

2. **Marinate:** In a bowl, mix together soy sauce, apple cider vinegar, honey (if using), ground ginger, minced garlic, and black pepper. Add the beef strips, ensuring they are well-coated. Marinate in the refrigerator for at least 2 hours, or overnight for deeper flavor.

3. **Oven Drying:** Preheat your oven to 175°F (80°C). Place marinated beef strips on a wire rack over a baking sheet. Bake for 4 hours, or until the jerky is dry and slightly chewy.

4. **Cool and Serve:** Allow the jerky to cool before transferring to an airtight container for storage.

Nutritional Information (per serving):

- Calories: 250
- Protein: 40g
- Fat: 7g
- Carbohydrates: 3g (without honey)
- Cholesterol: 105mg
- Sodium: 1,050mg

Chef's Tips:

- Removing as much fat as possible from the beef before slicing ensures a longer shelf life for the jerky.
- For a smokier flavor, you can add a pinch of smoked paprika to the marinade.
- Make sure the jerky cools completely before storing to prevent moisture from softening the jerky.

Spicy Chipotle Beef Jerky

Prep Time: 1 hour (for slicing and marinating)
Cook Time: 4 hours
Total Time: 5 hours
Servings: 6

Ingredients:

- 2 lbs lean beef (top round is ideal)
- 1/4 cup Worcestershire sauce
- 2 chipotle peppers in adobo sauce, finely chopped
- 1 tablespoon adobo sauce (from the chipotle peppers can)
- 1 teaspoon garlic powder
- 1 teaspoon onion powder
- 1 teaspoon sea salt
- 1/2 teaspoon cracked black pepper

Instructions:

1. **Prepare the Beef:** Freeze the beef slightly for easy slicing. Cut the beef into thin strips, about 1/8-inch thick, against the grain.

2. **Marinate:** Combine Worcestershire sauce, chopped chipotle peppers, adobo sauce, garlic powder, onion powder, sea salt, and black pepper in a mixing bowl. Add the beef strips, mixing well to coat. Marinate in the refrigerator for at least 1 hour or up to overnight.

3. **Dry the Beef:** Preheat the oven to 175°F (80°C). Arrange the beef strips on a wire rack set over a baking sheet. Ensure the strips do not overlap for even drying.

4. **Bake:** Place in the oven and bake for about 4 hours, or until the jerky is dry but still pliable.

5. **Cool and Store:** Let the jerky cool completely before storing in an airtight container.

Nutritional Information (per serving):

- Calories: 255
- Protein: 41g
- Fat: 8g
- Carbohydrates: 2g
- Cholesterol: 100mg
- Sodium: 1,100mg

Chef's Tips:

- Adjust the number of chipotle peppers to suit your spice preference. More peppers will increase the heat.

- Ensure the beef strips are fully submerged in the marinade for the most flavor.

- To keep jerky for an extended period, vacuum seal portions and store in a cool, dry place or the refrigerator.

Pork Rinds - How to puff and season at home.

Classic Salted Pork Rinds

Prep Time: 10 minutes (plus overnight drying)
Cook Time: 2 hours
Total Time: About 2 hours 10 minutes (plus overnight drying)
Servings: 6

Ingredients:

- 1 lb raw pork skin
- 2 tablespoons sea salt

Instructions:

1. **Prepare the Pork Skin:** Cut the pork skin into 2-inch squares. Place the pieces in a large pot of boiling water and cook for 1 hour to soften. Remove and pat dry. Lay the pieces on a baking sheet and refrigerate overnight to dry out.

2. **Oven Drying:** Preheat your oven to 200°F (93°C). Place the dried pork skin pieces on a baking sheet in a single layer. Bake for about 2 hours, or until they are completely dried out but not browned.

3. **Puffing:** Heat vegetable oil in a deep fryer or large pot to 400°F (204°C). Fry the pork skins in batches

until they puff up and become crispy, about 1 minute per batch. Remove with a slotted spoon and drain on paper towels.

4. **Season:** While still warm, sprinkle the pork rinds with sea salt.

5. **Serve:** Enjoy your homemade pork rinds as a crunchy, savory snack.

Nutritional Information (per serving):

- Calories: 150
- Protein: 17g
- Fat: 8g
- Carbohydrates: 0g
- Cholesterol: 45mg
- Sodium: 2,330mg

Chef's Tips:

- Ensure the pork skins are completely dry before frying to achieve the perfect puffiness.
- Adjust the salt according to your taste preference; you can also experiment with other seasonings like smoked paprika or garlic powder for variety.

- Store leftover pork rinds in an airtight container at room temperature to keep them crispy.

Spicy Chili Lime Pork Rinds

Prep Time: 10 minutes (plus overnight drying)
Cook Time: 2 hours
Total Time: About 2 hours 10 minutes (plus overnight drying)
Servings: 6

Ingredients:

- 1 lb raw pork skin
- 1 tablespoon chili powder
- 1 teaspoon lime zest
- 1 teaspoon sea salt
- 1/2 teaspoon cayenne pepper (adjust to taste)

Instructions:

1. **Prepare the Pork Skin:** Cut the pork skin into 2-inch pieces. Boil in water for 1 hour until soft. Pat dry, then place on a baking sheet. Refrigerate overnight to dry completely.

2. **Dry the Skins:** Preheat the oven to 200°F (93°C). Bake the dried pork skins for 2 hours until they are fully dried but not colored.

3. **Fry the Skins:** In a deep fryer or large pot, heat oil to 400°F (204°C). Fry the skins in small batches until they puff up, about 1 minute. Remove and drain on paper towels.

4. **Season:** Mix the chili powder, lime zest, sea salt, and cayenne pepper in a bowl. Sprinkle this mixture over the warm pork rinds and toss to coat evenly.

5. **Enjoy:** Serve the spicy chili lime pork rinds immediately, or store in an airtight container once cooled.

Nutritional Information (per serving):

- Calories: 152
- Protein: 17g
- Fat: 9g
- Carbohydrates: 1g
- Cholesterol: 46mg
- Sodium: 393mg

Chef's Tips:

- The lime zest adds a tangy kick that balances the heat from the chili and cayenne pepper. For best results, use fresh lime zest.

- Be careful when frying the pork skins; they should puff almost immediately. If not, the oil may not be hot enough.

- These pork rinds are perfect for dipping in guacamole or salsa for an extra flavor boost.

Smoky BBQ Pork Rinds

Prep Time: 10 minutes (plus overnight drying)
Cook Time: 2 hours
Total Time: About 2 hours 10 minutes (plus overnight drying)
Servings: 6

Ingredients:

- 1 lb raw pork skin
- 1 tablespoon smoked paprika
- 1 teaspoon garlic powder
- 1 teaspoon onion powder
- 1/2 teaspoon ground cumin
- 1/2 teaspoon sea salt
- 1/4 teaspoon black pepper

Instructions:

1. Prepare Pork Skin: Cut the pork skin into 2-inch squares. Boil in a large pot for 1 hour to soften. Drain, pat dry, and place on a baking sheet. Refrigerate overnight to further dry out.

2. Oven Drying: Preheat your oven to 200°F (93°C). Spread the pork skins on a baking sheet and bake for 2 hours, or until completely dried but not browned.

3. Deep Frying: Heat oil in a deep fryer or large pot to 400°F (204°C). Fry the pork skins in batches until they puff up and turn golden, about 1 minute per batch. Drain on paper towels.

4. Seasoning: Combine smoked paprika, garlic powder, onion powder, ground cumin, sea salt, and black pepper in a bowl. Sprinkle over the hot pork rinds and toss to coat evenly.

5. Serving: Enjoy the smoky BBQ pork rinds as a flavorful snack.

Nutritional Information (per serving):

- Calories: 153
- Protein: 17g
- Fat: 9g
- Carbohydrates: 2g
- Cholesterol: 47mg
- Sodium: 402mg

Chef's Tips:

- The key to crispy pork rinds is ensuring they are thoroughly dried before frying.
- Adjust the spice mix to suit your taste preferences. For extra heat, add a pinch of cayenne pepper.
- Store any leftovers in an airtight container to keep them crispy.

Parmesan & Herb Pork Rinds

Prep Time: 10 minutes (plus overnight drying)
Cook Time: 2 hours
Total Time: About 2 hours 10 minutes (plus overnight drying)
Servings: 6

Ingredients:

- 1 lb raw pork skin
- 1/4 cup grated Parmesan cheese
- 1 teaspoon dried oregano
- 1 teaspoon dried basil
- 1/2 teaspoon garlic powder
- Sea salt, to taste
- Olive oil spray (optional, for adherence of seasoning)

Instructions:

1. Prepare Pork Skin: Trim the pork skin into 2-inch pieces. Boil them for 1 hour until tender. Dry with paper towels, then refrigerate on a baking sheet overnight to dry out further.

2. Oven Drying: Set your oven to 200°F (93°C). Place the dried pork skins on a baking sheet and bake for 2 hours, or until fully dried but not colored.

3. Frying: Heat oil in a deep fryer to 400°F (204°C). Fry the pork skins in small batches until they puff up and become crispy, about 1 minute per batch. Drain on paper towels.

4. Season: Lightly spray the hot pork rinds with olive oil spray (if using). Mix the Parmesan, oregano, basil, garlic powder, and sea salt together and sprinkle over the pork rinds. Toss to evenly coat.

5. Enjoy: Serve the Parmesan & herb pork rinds immediately, or store them in an airtight container once they've cooled down.

Nutritional Information (per serving):

- Calories: 154
- Protein: 18g
- Fat: 9g
- Carbohydrates: 1g
- Cholesterol: 48mg
- Sodium: 403mg

Chef's Tips:

- The olive oil spray helps the seasoning stick to the pork rinds, but be careful not to make them soggy.
- These pork rinds are perfect as a standalone snack or can be crushed and used as a flavorful breadcrumb alternative for other dishes.
- For the best flavor, use high-quality Parmesan cheese and freshly ground herbs.

Appetizers Recipes

Classic Bacon-Wrapped Asparagus

Prep Time: 10 minutes
Cook Time: 20 minutes
Total Time: 30 minutes
Servings: 4

Ingredients:

- 16 asparagus spears, trimmed
- 8 slices of bacon
- Black pepper, to taste

Instructions:

1. **Preheat the Oven:** Set your oven to 400°F (200°C) and line a baking sheet with parchment paper for easy cleanup.

2. **Prepare the Asparagus:** Wash and trim the tough ends off the asparagus spears. If the spears are very thick, you might want to blanch them in boiling water for 1-2 minutes before wrapping with bacon.

3. **Wrap the Asparagus:** Cut the bacon slices in half lengthwise to create thin strips. Wrap each asparagus spear tightly with a strip of bacon,

starting from the bottom to just below the tip. Place the wrapped spears on the prepared baking sheet. Lightly season with black pepper.

4. **Bake:** Place in the preheated oven and bake for 20 minutes, or until the bacon is crispy and the asparagus is tender.

5. **Serve:** Enjoy these bacon-wrapped asparagus spears warm as a delicious and simple appetizer.

Nutritional Information (per serving):

- Calories: 180
- Protein: 10g
- Fat: 14g
- Carbohydrates: 4g
- Cholesterol: 25mg
- Sodium: 400mg

Chef's Tips:

- For extra flavor, you can sprinkle a little garlic powder or Parmesan cheese over the bacon-wrapped asparagus before baking.

- Turning the asparagus halfway through the cooking time can help ensure the bacon crisps up evenly.

- To keep the asparagus green and vibrant, consider blanching before wrapping with bacon. This step is optional but can enhance the texture and appearance.

Bacon-Wrapped Asparagus with Balsamic Glaze

Prep Time: 15 minutes
Cook Time: 25 minutes
Total Time: 40 minutes
Servings: 4

Ingredients:

- 16 asparagus spears, trimmed

- 8 slices of bacon

- 2 tablespoons balsamic vinegar reduction (optional for those strictly following a carnivore diet)

- Freshly ground black pepper, to taste

Instructions:

1. **Preheat Oven:** Heat your oven to 400°F (200°C). Prepare a baking sheet by lining it with parchment paper.

2. **Prepare Asparagus:** Clean the asparagus and trim away the woody ends. If desired, blanch the asparagus in boiling water for 1 minute, then transfer to an ice bath to stop the cooking process.

3. **Wrap with Bacon:** Wrap each asparagus spear with a half slice of bacon, starting from the bottom and spiraling up to just below the tip. Arrange the wrapped spears on the baking sheet. Season with black pepper.

4. **Bake:** Bake in the preheated oven for 20-25 minutes, or until the bacon is crispy. If using, brush the asparagus with balsamic reduction in the last 5 minutes of cooking.

5. **Serve:** Present the bacon-wrapped asparagus on a platter, optionally drizzled with more balsamic reduction.

Nutritional Information (per serving):

- Calories: 190
- Protein: 11g
- Fat: 15g
- Carbohydrates: 5g (excluding balsamic reduction)
- Cholesterol: 30mg
- Sodium: 420mg

Chef's Tips:

- The balsamic reduction adds a sweet and tangy flavor that complements the smokiness of the bacon; however, it can be omitted for a pure carnivore approach.
- For even cooking and crispiness, avoid overlapping the bacon when wrapping the asparagus.
- The asparagus can be prepared ahead of time and stored in the refrigerator until ready to bake, making this an easy appetizer for entertaining.

Bacon-Wrapped Asparagus with Lemon Pepper

Prep Time: 15 minutes
Cook Time: 20 minutes
Total Time: 35 minutes
Servings: 4

Ingredients:

- 16 asparagus spears, trimmed
- 8 slices of bacon
- 1 teaspoon lemon zest
- 1/2 teaspoon cracked black pepper
- Olive oil spray (optional)

Instructions:

1. **Preheat Oven:** Adjust your oven rack to the middle position and preheat to 400°F (200°C). Line a baking sheet with foil for easy cleanup and place a wire rack on top.

2. **Prepare Asparagus:** Lightly spray the asparagus spears with olive oil (if using). This helps the seasoning stick and promotes even cooking.

3. **Season:** In a small bowl, mix together lemon zest and cracked black pepper. Sprinkle this mixture over the asparagus spears.

4. **Wrap with Bacon:** Cut the bacon slices in half lengthwise to make them thinner. Wrap each seasoned asparagus spear with a strip of bacon, securing the ends. Arrange on the wire rack.

5. **Bake:** Bake for 20 minutes, or until the bacon is crispy and the asparagus is tender.

6. **Serve:** Offer these lemon pepper bacon-wrapped asparagus hot as a flavorful and refreshing appetizer.

Nutritional Information (per serving):

- Calories: 182
- Protein: 10g
- Fat: 14g
- Carbohydrates: 4g
- Cholesterol: 25mg
- Sodium: 402mg

Chef's Tips:

- The lemon zest adds a fresh and zesty flavor that cuts through the richness of the bacon.

- Placing the wrapped asparagus on a wire rack helps the bacon get crispy all around without needing to flip them during baking.

- For an added touch of lemon, you can squeeze a bit of lemon juice over the asparagus before serving.

Bacon-Wrapped Asparagus with Creamy Horseradish Dip

Prep Time: 20 minutes
Cook Time: 20 minutes
Total Time: 40 minutes
Servings: 4

Ingredients:

For the Asparagus:

- 16 asparagus spears, trimmed
- 8 slices of bacon
- Salt, to taste
- Freshly ground black pepper, to taste

For the Horseradish Dip:

- 1/2 cup sour cream
- 2 tablespoons prepared horseradish
- 1 teaspoon Dijon mustard
- Salt and pepper, to taste

Instructions:

1. **Preheat Oven:** Heat your oven to 400°F (200°C) and line a baking sheet with parchment paper or foil.
2. **Season Asparagus:** Lightly season the asparagus spears with salt and freshly ground black pepper.
3. **Wrap Asparagus:** Cut the bacon slices in half lengthwise and wrap each asparagus spear tightly with a piece of bacon. Place the wrapped spears on the prepared baking sheet.
4. **Bake:** Transfer to the oven and bake for 20 minutes, or until the bacon is crispy and the asparagus is tender.
5. **Prepare the Horseradish Dip:** While the asparagus bakes, mix together sour cream, horseradish, Dijon mustard, salt, and pepper in a small bowl. Adjust seasoning to taste.
6. **Serve:** Arrange the bacon-wrapped asparagus on a serving platter with the creamy horseradish dip on the side.

Nutritional Information (per serving):

- Calories: 198
- Protein: 11g

- Fat: 16g
- Carbohydrates: 5g
- Cholesterol: 30mg
- Sodium: 408mg

Chef's Tips:

- Blotting the bacon with paper towels before wrapping can help reduce grease and ensure a crispier finish.
- The creamy horseradish dip can be made in advance and stored in the refrigerator to allow the flavors to meld together.
- Adjust the amount of horseradish in the dip according to your preference for spiciness.

Top of Form Scallops seared in Ghee - Light and rich in flavor.

Classic Seared Scallops in Ghee with Lemon Zest

Prep Time: 5 minutes
Cook Time: 6 minutes
Total Time: 11 minutes
Servings: 4

Ingredients:

- 12 large sea scallops, patted dry
- 2 tablespoons ghee
- Zest of 1 lemon (optional for those strictly following a carnivore diet)
- Salt and freshly ground black pepper, to taste

Instructions:

1. **Prepare Scallops:** Ensure scallops are dry by patting them with paper towels. Season both sides with salt and pepper.
2. **Heat Pan:** In a large skillet, heat the ghee over medium-high heat until hot but not smoking.

3. **Sear Scallops:** Add the scallops to the pan, making sure not to overcrowd. Cook for about 3 minutes on one side until a golden crust forms. Flip and cook for an additional 2-3 minutes on the other side.

4. **Serve:** Remove the scallops from the pan and arrange on a serving platter. Sprinkle with lemon zest for added flavor (if using). Serve immediately.

Nutritional Information (per serving):

- Calories: 120
- Protein: 14g
- Fat: 6g
- Carbohydrates: 2g (0g if not using lemon zest)
- Cholesterol: 27mg
- Sodium: 350mg

Chef's Tips:

- Ensure scallops are completely dry before searing to achieve a perfect crust.
- Avoid moving the scallops around once they hit the pan to allow a golden crust to form.

- The addition of lemon zest adds a fresh, bright flavor that complements the richness of the ghee, but it can be omitted for a strict carnivore approach.

Garlic Herb Seared Scallops in Ghee

Prep Time: 5 minutes
Cook Time: 6 minutes
Total Time: 11 minutes
Servings: 4

Ingredients:

- 12 large sea scallops, patted dry
- 2 tablespoons ghee
- 1 teaspoon garlic powder (optional for those strictly following a carnivore diet)
- 1 teaspoon dried parsley
- Salt and freshly ground black pepper, to taste

Instructions:

1. **Prepare Scallops:** Dry the scallops thoroughly with paper towels and season with salt, pepper, garlic powder (if using), and dried parsley.

2. **Heat Ghee:** In a skillet over medium-high heat, melt the ghee until shimmering.

3. **Cook Scallops:** Place scallops in the pan in a single layer. Sear without moving them for about 3 minutes or until a golden crust forms. Flip the scallops and cook for an additional 2-3 minutes.

4. **Serve:** Transfer the scallops to a serving dish. They can be garnished with additional parsley if desired. Serve hot.

Nutritional Information (per serving):

- Calories: 122
- Protein: 14g
- Fat: 6g
- Carbohydrates: 1g (0g if not using garlic powder)
- Cholesterol: 27mg
- Sodium: 352mg

Chef's Tips:

- To ensure even cooking, do not overcrowd the pan; cook in batches if necessary.

- The use of garlic powder and dried parsley is optional and can be tailored to fit a strict carnivore diet.

- For those not strictly following a carnivore diet, a squeeze of lemon juice can be added just before serving for a zesty finish.

Spicy Cajun Seared Scallops in Ghee

Prep Time: 5 minutes
Cook Time: 6 minutes
Total Time: 11 minutes
Servings: 4

Ingredients:

- 12 large sea scallops, patted dry
- 2 tablespoons ghee
- 1 teaspoon Cajun seasoning (ensure it's free of additives for a strict carnivore diet)
- Salt, to taste

Instructions:

1. **Season Scallops:** Lightly season the dry scallops with Cajun seasoning and a pinch of salt.
2. **Heat Ghee:** In a heavy skillet, heat the ghee over medium-high heat until it's shimmering but not smoking.
3. **Sear Scallops:** Place the scallops in the skillet, making sure not to overcrowd them. Sear for about 3 minutes on one side until a golden crust forms,

then flip and sear for another 2-3 minutes on the other side until cooked through and golden.

4. **Serve:** Immediately transfer the scallops to a serving plate. For those not strictly adhering to a carnivore diet, a squeeze of lemon juice can enhance the flavors.

Nutritional Information (per serving):

- Calories: 123
- Protein: 14g
- Fat: 7g
- Carbohydrates: 1g
- Cholesterol: 27mg
- Sodium: 360mg

Chef's Tips:

- Make sure the scallops are completely dry before seasoning to ensure proper searing.
- Adjust the amount of Cajun seasoning based on your spice preference.
- Serve immediately to enjoy the scallops at their best texture and flavor.

Herb-Butter Seared Scallops in Ghee

Prep Time: 10 minutes
Cook Time: 6 minutes
Total Time: 16 minutes
Servings: 4

Ingredients:

- 12 large sea scallops, patted dry
- 2 tablespoons ghee
- 1 tablespoon unsalted butter
- 1 teaspoon dried herbs (such as thyme or rosemary)
- Salt and freshly ground black pepper, to taste

Instructions:

1. **Prepare Scallops:** Season the scallops with salt, pepper, and dried herbs.

2. **Melt Ghee and Butter:** In a skillet over medium-high heat, melt the ghee together with the unsalted butter.

3. **Sear Scallops:** Once the ghee and butter mixture is hot, add the scallops. Sear them for about 3 minutes on one side until they develop a crust. Flip

the scallops and cook for an additional 2-3 minutes until they are opaque and cooked through.

4. **Serve:** Remove the scallops from the skillet and arrange them on a warm plate. They can be garnished with additional herbs if desired.

Nutritional Information (per serving):

- Calories: 125
- Protein: 14g
- Fat: 8g
- Carbohydrates: 0g
- Cholesterol: 30mg
- Sodium: 370mg

Chef's Tips:

- Avoid moving the scallops around in the pan to ensure they develop a nice, golden crust.
- Combining ghee with a bit of butter adds a rich, nutty flavor that complements the natural sweetness of the scallops.
- Choose high-quality, dry-packed scallops for the best searing results and flavor.

Mini Meatballs with Spicy Dipping Sauce - A crowd-pleaser, perfect for entertaining.

Classic Mini Meatballs with Creamy Sriracha Sauce

Prep Time: 15 minutes
Cook Time: 20 minutes
Total Time: 35 minutes
Servings: 6

Ingredients:

For the Mini Meatballs:

- 1 lb ground beef (85% lean)
- 1 lb ground pork
- 2 teaspoons sea salt
- 1 teaspoon black pepper
- 1 teaspoon garlic powder
- 1 teaspoon onion powder

For the Creamy Sriracha Sauce:

- 1/2 cup mayonnaise (choose a brand with no added sugar)
- 2 tablespoons Sriracha sauce (adjust based on heat preference)
- 1 tablespoon apple cider vinegar

Instructions:

1. **Preheat Oven:** Set your oven to 400°F (200°C) and line a baking sheet with parchment paper.
2. **Mix Meatball Ingredients:** In a large bowl, combine ground beef, ground pork, sea salt, black pepper, garlic powder, and onion powder. Mix until just combined, being careful not to overmix.
3. **Form Mini Meatballs:** Shape the mixture into small, bite-sized meatballs, about 1 inch in diameter, and place them on the prepared baking sheet.
4. **Bake Meatballs:** Bake in the preheated oven for 18-20 minutes, or until the meatballs are cooked through and browned on the outside.
5. **Prepare Creamy Sriracha Sauce:** While the meatballs are baking, whisk together mayonnaise, Sriracha sauce, and apple cider vinegar in a small bowl until smooth.
6. **Serve:** Serve the mini meatballs hot with the creamy Sriracha sauce on the side for dipping.

Nutritional Information (per serving):

- Calories: 320
- Protein: 24g
- Fat: 24g
- Carbohydrates: 1g
- Cholesterol: 80mg
- Sodium: 800mg

Chef's Tips:

- Avoid packing the meatballs too tightly when forming them to ensure they remain tender after baking.
- The creamy Sriracha sauce can be made in advance and stored in the refrigerator to allow the flavors to meld.
- For a smoother dipping sauce, blend the sauce ingredients together in a food processor or blender.

Herbed Mini Meatballs with Spicy Mustard Dipping Sauce

Prep Time: 15 minutes
Cook Time: 20 minutes
Total Time: 35 minutes
Servings: 6

Ingredients:

For the Mini Meatballs:

- 1 lb ground lamb
- 1 lb ground beef (90% lean)
- 2 teaspoons sea salt
- 1 teaspoon dried oregano
- 1 teaspoon dried basil
- 1/2 teaspoon cracked black pepper

For the Spicy Mustard Dipping Sauce:

- 1/2 cup Dijon mustard
- 2 tablespoons hot sauce (adjust to taste)
- 1 teaspoon Worcestershire sauce (ensure it's a version without added sugar)

Instructions:

1. **Preheat Oven:** Heat your oven to 400°F (200°C). Prepare a baking sheet with parchment paper.
2. **Combine Meatball Ingredients:** In a mixing bowl, blend together the ground lamb, ground

beef, sea salt, oregano, basil, and black pepper. Mix until evenly combined.
3. **Form Mini Meatballs:** Roll the mixture into small meatballs, approximately 1 inch in diameter, and arrange them on the baking sheet.
4. **Bake:** Place the meatballs in the oven and bake for 18-20 minutes, or until they're fully cooked and have a nice exterior browning.
5. **Make Spicy Mustard Sauce:** While the meatballs bake, mix Dijon mustard, hot sauce, and Worcestershire sauce in a bowl until combined.
6. **Serve:** Offer the baked mini meatballs with the spicy mustard dipping sauce on the side.

Nutritional Information (per serving):

- Calories: 330
- Protein: 26g
- Fat: 23g
- Carbohydrates: 2g
- Cholesterol: 85mg
- Sodium: 870mg

Chef's Tips:

- Gently mix the meatball ingredients to avoid overworking the meat, which can result in tough meatballs.
- The spicy mustard dipping sauce's heat level can be adjusted by increasing or decreasing the amount of hot sauce.

- These mini meatballs and sauce can be prepared ahead of time, making them perfect for entertaining. Reheat the meatballs in the oven before serving to ensure they are warm and juicy.

Asian-Inspired Mini Meatballs with Ginger Soy Dipping Sauce

Prep Time: 20 minutes
Cook Time: 20 minutes
Total Time: 40 minutes
Servings: 6

Ingredients:

For the Mini Meatballs:

- 1 lb ground chicken
- 1 lb ground turkey
- 2 teaspoons sea salt
- 1 teaspoon ground ginger
- 1 teaspoon garlic powder
- 1/2 teaspoon black pepper
- 2 green onions, finely chopped

For the Ginger Soy Dipping Sauce:

- 1/4 cup soy sauce (use a low-sodium, gluten-free version if preferred)
- 2 tablespoons rice vinegar
- 1 tablespoon honey (omit for a strict carnivore diet or use a carnivore-approved sweetener)
- 1 teaspoon sesame oil
- 1 tablespoon fresh ginger, minced
- 1 clove garlic, minced
- Red pepper flakes, to taste

Instructions:

1. **Prepare the Meatballs:** In a large bowl, combine ground chicken, ground turkey, sea salt, ground ginger, garlic powder, black pepper, and green onions. Mix until well blended.
2. **Form Mini Meatballs:** Shape the mixture into small, bite-sized meatballs, about 1 inch in diameter, and place them on a lined baking sheet.
3. **Bake Meatballs:** Preheat the oven to 400°F (200°C). Bake the meatballs for 20 minutes, or until cooked through and lightly golden on the outside.
4. **Make the Dipping Sauce:** While the meatballs are baking, whisk together soy sauce, rice vinegar, honey (if using), sesame oil, minced ginger, minced garlic, and red pepper flakes in a small bowl. Adjust seasoning to taste.
5. **Serve:** Arrange the cooked meatballs on a platter and serve with the ginger soy dipping sauce on the side.

Nutritional Information (per serving):

- Calories: 280
- Protein: 26g
- Fat: 16g
- Carbohydrates: 5g (less if honey is omitted)
- Cholesterol: 98mg
- Sodium: 800mg

Chef's Tips:

- Ensure the meat mixture is thoroughly combined for uniform flavor and texture in each meatball.
- Baking on a wire rack over a baking sheet can help the meatballs cook evenly and become slightly crisp on the outside.
- The ginger soy dipping sauce can be made ahead of time and stored in the refrigerator to enhance its flavors.

Southwest Mini Meatballs with Chipotle Adobo Sauce

Prep Time: 15 minutes
Cook Time: 20 minutes
Total Time: 35 minutes
Servings: 6

Ingredients:

For the Mini Meatballs:

- 1 lb ground beef (85% lean)
- 1 lb ground pork
- 2 teaspoons sea salt
- 1 teaspoon cumin
- 1 teaspoon smoked paprika
- 1/2 teaspoon garlic powder
- 1/2 teaspoon onion powder
- 1/4 teaspoon chili powder

For the Chipotle Adobo Sauce:

- 1/2 cup mayonnaise
- 2 chipotle peppers in adobo sauce, finely chopped
- 1 tablespoon adobo sauce (from the chipotle peppers)
- 1 teaspoon lime juice
- Salt, to taste

Instructions:

1. **Prepare the Meatballs:** In a mixing bowl, combine the ground beef, ground pork, sea salt, cumin, smoked paprika, garlic powder, onion powder, and chili powder. Mix until just combined.
2. **Form Mini Meatballs:** Roll the mixture into small meatballs, about 1 inch in diameter, and place them on a parchment-lined baking tray.
3. **Bake Meatballs:** Preheat the oven to 400°F (200°C). Bake the meatballs for 20 minutes, or until they are browned and cooked through.
4. **Make the Chipotle Adobo Sauce:** While the meatballs are baking, mix together mayonnaise, chopped chipotle peppers, adobo sauce, and lime juice in a bowl. Season with salt to taste.
5. **Serve:** Serve the hot mini meatballs with the chipotle adobo sauce for dipping.

Nutritional Information (per serving):

- Calories: 320
- Protein: 24g
- Fat: 24g
- Carbohydrates: 2g
- Cholesterol: 85mg
- Sodium: 1,020mg

Chef's Tips:

- Mixing the meats by hand until just combined ensures the meatballs remain tender and juicy.
- The chipotle adobo sauce can be adjusted for heat by adding more or less of the chipotle peppers and adobo sauce.
- For a smoother dipping sauce, the ingredients can be blended until smooth, adjusting the

Weekly Structure:

Day 1:

- Breakfast: Classic Steak and Eggs
- Lunch: Crispy Chicken Skins
- Dinner: Seared Salmon with Herb Butter

Day 2:

- Breakfast: Bacon and Mushroom Omelette
- Lunch: Carnivore Diet Beef Jerky (as a snack or part of a meal)
- Dinner: Roast Chicken with Ghee and Spices

Day 3:

- Breakfast: Pork Belly and Eggs
- Lunch: Tuna Salad with Homemade Mayo
- Dinner: Lamb Chops with Rosemary Butter

Day 4:

- Breakfast: Chicken Liver Pâté on Pork Rinds
- Lunch: Sardines or Mackerel with Avocado (for those including it in their carnivore diet)

- Dinner: Beef Ribeye with Bone Marrow Butter

Day 5:

- Breakfast: Smoked Salmon with Cream Cheese
- Lunch: Cold Cuts with Cheese Slices (for a light meal)
- Dinner: Slow-Cooked Pork Shoulder

Day 6:

- Breakfast: Scrambled Eggs with Diced Ham
- Lunch: Bacon-Wrapped Asparagus
- Dinner: Grilled Trout with Lemon Butter

Day 7:

- Breakfast: Beef Liver Fried with Onions
- Lunch: Chicken Thighs with Skin, Baked
- Dinner: Venison Steaks with a Side of Bone Broth

Notes for the Meal Plan:

- **Variety:** Each week, rotate the types of meat and fish to include beef, pork, chicken, lamb, fish, and organ meats to ensure a range of nutrients.

- **Cooking Methods:** Utilize various cooking methods like grilling, roasting, slow cooking, and pan-searing to diversify flavors and textures.

- **Seasonings:** Use simple seasonings like salt, pepper, and herbs. Ensure any added fats are from high-quality sources like ghee, butter, or animal fats.

- **Adjustments:** Feel free to swap meals between days to suit preferences and availability. The key is maintaining variety and nutritional balance.

- **Leftovers:** Strategically plan to cook in batches where leftovers can serve as the next day's lunch, saving time and effort.

Implementing the Plan:

- **Shopping List:** Based on the weekly plan, create a shopping list that covers all the meats, eggs, and any additional items like high-quality dairy or specific fats needed for cooking and seasoning.

- **Preparation:** Some meals can be prepped in advance, especially breakfasts and lunches. Consider preparing meats or bases that can be used in multiple meals throughout the week.

- **Flexibility:** The beauty of a carnivore diet lies in its simplicity. Feel free to repeat favorite meals and adjust portions based on hunger and nutritional needs.

Meats:

- Beef: Ribeye steaks, ground beef, beef liver, brisket
- Pork: Pork belly, pork shoulder, bacon, pork chops
- Chicken: Whole chickens, chicken thighs (skin-on), chicken breasts, chicken liver
- Lamb: Lamb chops, ground lamb
- Fish and Seafood: Salmon, trout, sardines, mackerel, shrimp, scallops
- Other: Venison, duck breasts

Dairy (optional, based on dietary preferences):

- Butter (preferably grass-fed)
- Heavy cream
- Hard cheeses (e.g., Parmesan, aged cheddar)
- Cream cheese

Fats and Oils:

- Ghee
- Lard
- Duck fat

- Tallow

Seasonings (optional, for those not strictly carnivore):

- Sea salt
- Black pepper
- Garlic powder
- Onion powder
- Herbs: Rosemary, thyme, oregano (fresh or dried)
- Spices: Paprika, cayenne pepper, chili powder

Weekly Meal Planner Template

Monday:

- Breakfast: Scrambled eggs with diced bacon
- Lunch: Grilled chicken salad (chicken, mixed greens for keto-carnivore, olive oil)
- Dinner: Ribeye steak with sautéed mushrooms in butter
- Snack: Pork rinds

Tuesday:

- Breakfast: Bacon and eggs
- Lunch: Leftover ribeye steak, cold, with hard cheese slices
- Dinner: Baked salmon with lemon butter sauce
- Snack: Beef jerky

Wednesday:

- Breakfast: Chicken liver fried with onions (for those including some vegetables)
- Lunch: Tuna salad with mayonnaise
- Dinner: Slow-cooked pork shoulder
- Snack: Hard-boiled eggs

Thursday:

- Breakfast: Omelet with cheese and ham
- Lunch: Cold cuts with cheese and a handful of nuts (for keto-carnivore)
- Dinner: Lamb chops with rosemary and garlic
- Snack: Cheese sticks

Friday:

- Breakfast: Fried eggs with side of avocado (keto-carnivore)
- Lunch: Shredded chicken mixed with cream cheese and herbs
- Dinner: Grilled trout with a side of asparagus wrapped in bacon
- Snack: Smoked salmon with cream cheese

Saturday:

- Breakfast: Liver pate on pork rinds
- Lunch: Beef meatballs with spicy dipping sauce
- Dinner: Duck breast with a side of sautéed spinach (for those including some vegetables)
- Snack: Sliced hard cheese

Sunday:

- Breakfast: Pancakes made from cream cheese and eggs, served with butter (for a more flexible diet)
- Lunch: Roast beef slices with horseradish cream
- Dinner: Grilled shrimp with garlic butter

- Snack: Deviled eggs

Tips for Using the Templates:

- **Flexibility:** Adjust the meal planner based on your calorie needs, dietary goals, and any intolerances. Feel free to swap meals and days to fit your schedule.

- **Batch Cooking:** Consider preparing larger quantities of meats to have ready-to-eat proteins on hand, saving time throughout the week.

- **Quality Over Quantity:** Focus on sourcing the best quality animal products you can afford, emphasizing grass-fed, pasture-raised, and wild-caught options.

- **Seasoning:** Use seasonings sparingly if you're strictly carnivore but feel free to add variety with approved spices if you're more flexible.

- **Hydration:** Remember to stay hydrated, primarily drinking water. Bone broth is also a great option for additional nutrients and electrolytes.

Printed in Great Britain
by Amazon